THE ALCHEMY OF HEALING

MASTER ANCIENT HAWAIIAN TECHNIQUE, CRUSH NEGATIVE EMOTIONS, TRANSFORM SUBCONSCIOUS PATTERNS, AND SELF-HEAL YOUR WAY TO A HOLISTIC LIFESTYLE

SOORAJ ACHAR

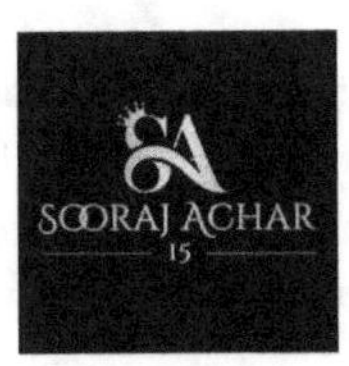

WWW.SOORAJACHAR.COM

YOUR FREE GIFT

As a token of my thanks for taking out time to read my book, I would like to offer you a **Free-Gift**:

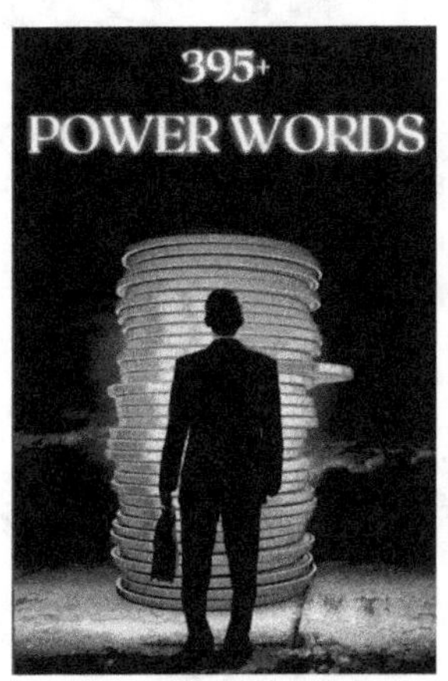

Scan the QR Code below to Download your **Free eBook PDF**.

Learn 395+ Surprising Psychology Words That Will Change The Way You Think - in the Next 30 Days!

You can also grab your **FREE GIFT** by typing in the below URL: **https://gift.sooraj-achar.com/**

ABOUT AUTHOR

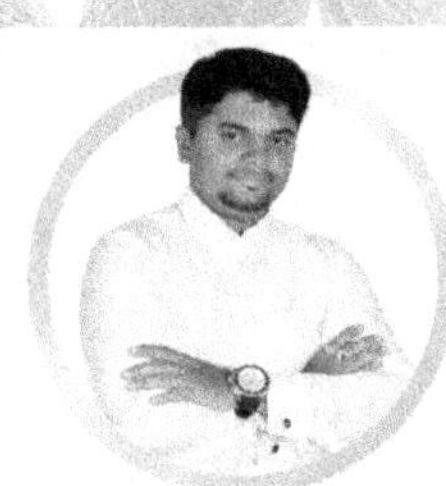

Sooraj Achar, the Accomplished Author of **"The Alchemy of Healing"** - A Sensational #1 Bestseller Across the Globe

Dive into the world of **Sooraj Achar**, a prodigious author hailing from Bangalore, India, whose exceptional journey is as intriguing as the profound concepts explored in his works. With **"The Ultimate Self-Healing Mastery Series,"** Sooraj has transcended borders, achieving the coveted status of **#1 Bestseller** in the United States, the United Kingdom, Canada, India, and Australia.

A Remarkable Beginnings:

Sooraj Achar's extraordinary odyssey commenced in the vibrant city of Bangalore, India. As a young dreamer, his fascination with mathematics sparked an early connection with the enigmatic world of numbers. This infatuation, initially drawn from captivating numerological stories, sowed the seeds for a lifetime dedicated to the exploration of **Numerical Mysteries**.

A Multifaceted Expert:

Today, **Sooraj Achar** stands as not just an accomplished Software Engineer but also a passionate connoisseur of **numerology** and the ancient science of **Feng-Shui (Vastu)**. His multifaceted persona extends to **coaching and consulting**, where he delves into the profound questions of Health, Relationships, Careers, and Money (HRCM). Sooraj is a certified **Ho'oponopono & EFT Healer and NLP Practitioner**, renowned for his transformative abilities in bringing about balance, harmony, and fulfillment in the lives of countless individuals.

A Seeker of Wisdom:

Sooraj's relentless quest for knowledge has led him to the intricate realms of human psychology and behavior. His dedication to understanding the human psyche and optimizing life's potential is unwavering. As a perpetual learner, he embodies the principles of optimal living and shares his wisdom to empower others to lead resourceful lives.

A Believer in Unlimited Potential:

Above all, **Sooraj Achar** is a firm believer in the limitless potential residing within each individual. He ardently champions the idea that every person possesses the capacity to achieve far beyond their self-imposed limits. Through his words and wisdom, he inspires others to unlock their hidden potential and lead lives of purpose and abundance.

For more life-altering insights, delve into Sooraj Achar's remarkable catalog of books. Visit www.sooraj-achar.com and embark on a journey of self-discovery and transformation.

Stay Connected:

Explore the latest updates, thought-provoking content, and inspiring messages from Sooraj Achar by connecting with him through our social media channels. Join us in the pursuit of a fulfilling and harmonious life.

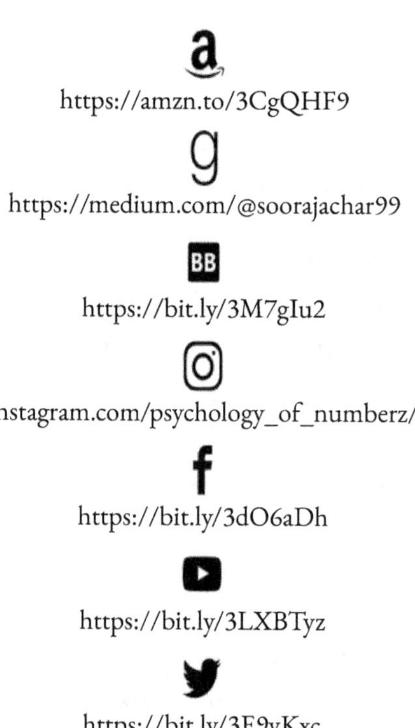

ACKNOWLEDGEMENTS

How does a person say **"Thank You"** when there are so many people to thank?

Obviously, this book is a big thank you to my father **G Sathyanarayan Achar,** who is a powerful role model, and my mother **G Pramila,** who taught me love and kindness.

I extend my heartfelt appreciation to my sister, **Shruthi S**, brother-in-law, **Saravana P**, and adorable niece, **Naveeksha S**, who have played pivotal roles in making this book a reality. Their presence makes my life complete.

My mentor, **Mr. Mitesh Khatri,** deserves a special acknowledgment for teaching and guiding me to become a **certified healer** in **Ho'Oponopono & EFT**.

I owe thanks to **Mr. Som Bathla,** an **Amazon #1 Bestselling** author, for his mentorship, motivation, and guidance in the realms of **Writing, Self-Publishing, and Launching Books**. His support has been instrumental in initiating my journey as an Authorpreneur.

Finally, heartfelt gratitude to my dedicated team – **Avesh Ansari**, **Akshay Bhat**, and **Md. Bilal** – for their unwavering support and contributions.

DEDICATION

This Book is Dedicated to My Grandparents,

R. Gangadhar & G. Vishalakshamma

And, My Dear Brother **Arvind Achar.**

CONTENTS

HOW THIS BOOK CAN WORK MIRACLES IN YOUR LIFE?

"The four phrases of Ho'Oponopono are the keys to unlock the doors of your heart and set yourself free."

– Dr. Joe Vitale

In the tapestry of ancient wisdom, there exists a profound art of healing, a timeless technique rooted in the heart of Hawaiian traditions. "The Alchemy of Healing" is not just a book; it's a transformative guide that invites you on a journey to master the ancient Hawaiian technique of Ho'oponopono. This technique, often hailed as a catalyst for miracles, unveils a path to crush negative emotions, transform subconscious patterns, and embark on a journey of self-healing toward a holistic life.

Illuminate Your Inner Alchemy:

At the core of this transformative journey is the illumination of your inner alchemy. Ho'oponopono, a term that translates to "to make right," becomes your guiding light. Through the pages of this book, you'll unravel the mysteries of this ancient practice, understanding how it has been a sacred key to healing in Hawaiian culture for generations. The book serves as a gateway, introducing you to the profound art of healing within, a journey that is both enlightening and empowering.

Crush Negative Emotions:

Negative emotions can act as heavy anchors, weighing down our spirits and hindering our progress. "The Alchemy of Healing" empowers you with the tools to crush these emotional burdens through the transformative power of Ho'oponopono. As you delve into the practical applications of this ancient technique, you'll learn to dissolve negativity and free yourself from the chains of emotional turmoil. This section becomes your compass, guiding you toward emotional liberation and a newfound sense of lightness.

Transform Subconscious Patterns:

The subconscious mind holds the blueprints of our habits and patterns, many of which operate beneath our conscious awareness. In this book, you'll embark on a profound exploration of your subconscious, unraveling patterns that may have been woven into the fabric of your being. Through the alchemical principles of Ho'oponopono, you'll learn to transform these patterns, rewriting the script of your life and fostering a narrative of empowerment and resilience.

Self-Heal Your Way to a Holistic Life:

Holistic healing is a journey that encompasses the mind, body, and spirit. "The Alchemy of Healing" provides a comprehensive roadmap for self-healing that goes beyond surface-level solutions. Through the wisdom of Ho'oponopono, you'll tap into your innate healing powers, addressing physical, emotional, and spiritual dimensions of your being. This section becomes a sanctuary, offering you practical tools to cultivate a holistic life that radiates well-being.

Experience Miracles Unfolding:

As you integrate the principles of Ho'oponopono into your daily life, be prepared to witness miracles unfold. This isn't about wishful thinking; it's about aligning yourself with the natural flow of the universe. From improved relationships to enhanced well-being, the transformative power of this ancient technique opens the door to positive shifts that might leave you awe-inspired.

Embrace Holistic Wellness:

Holistic wellness is the harmonious integration of mind, body, and spirit. "The Alchemy of Healing" guides you to embrace this wellness through the principles of Ho'oponopono. This isn't a one-size-fits-all approach; instead, it encourages you to tailor the practice to your unique needs. As you apply the teachings, you'll find yourself on a journey toward a life where every aspect resonates with harmony, fostering a profound sense of peace and vitality.

Manifest Your Desires:

The alchemy of healing isn't just about addressing challenges; it's also about co-creating the reality you desire. In this segment of the book, you'll delve into the art of manifestation through Ho'oponopono. The ancient Hawaiians believed that aligning your intentions with the universal flow could lead to effortless manifestation. "The Alchemy of Healing" empowers you to understand this art, guiding you to manifest your desires with clarity and purpose.

"The Alchemy of Healing" isn't just a guide; it's an invitation to transform your life on every level. Through the ancient wisdom of Ho'oponopono, you'll discover the profound art of healing that has been revered for centuries. This book is your companion on a journey of self-discovery, empowerment, and healing. The alchemy of miracles awaits—immerse yourself in the transformative power of Ho'oponopono and start rewriting the story of your life today.

CHAPTER HIGHLIGHTS: TOP 5 TAKEAWAYS AND INSIGHTS

1. Key Takeaways from the chapter - Soulful Cleansing: Embracing Ho'Oponopono For Inner Harmony:

1. Ho'Oponopono Technique's Healing Power: Dr. Hew Len's Ho'Oponopono technique healed violent patients without medicine or direct contact, showcasing its extraordinary power at an energy level.

2. Words' Frequency Impact: The four statements - "I am sorry, please forgive me, thank you, I love you" - hold powerful frequency vibrations that can clear negative energy between individuals.

3. Energy-Level Communication: The technique teaches how to connect and communicate with others at the energy level, influencing positive change without physical interaction.

4. Rules for Effective Practice: Follow rules like closing your eyes, allowing emotions, and maintaining zero body movement during the technique to enhance its effectiveness.

5. Comprehensive Exercise Steps: The step-by-step exercises involve apologizing, forgiving, and expressing love to others, including oneself, promoting emotional release and inner healing.

2. Key Takeaways from the chapter - Understanding The Basics: Ho'Oponopono Demystified:

1. Total Responsibility Empowers Transformation: Ho'Oponopono is about taking 100% responsibility for every aspect of your life. By doing so, you regain the power to heal and transform your circumstances.

2. Miraculous Healing Power: The chapter narrates a remarkable story of an Indian Air Force Commander who, against medical odds, healed and returned to flying through dedicated Ho'Oponopono practice.

3. Positive Crazy Goals Over Negative Realistic Goals: Encourages setting positive, ambitious goals over negative, realistic ones. The story exemplifies how embracing a positive crazy goal led to a miraculous outcome.

4. Logic Hinders Magic: To navigate the magical world we inhabit, the key rule is to avoid relying on logic based on past experiences. Ho'Oponopono serves as a tool to overcome the limitations of logic and create a future unbound by the past.

5. Basic and Advanced Ho'Oponopono: Distinguishes between basic Ho'Oponopono for external matters and advanced Ho'Oponopono for self-healing. Provides a simple 108-times practice for external issues and emphasizes unconditional practice for its effectiveness. introduces walking-talking Ho'Oponopono for instant healing throughout the day.

3. Key Takeaways from the chapter - Beyond Basics: Advanced Ho'Oponopono Mastery:

1. Advanced Ho'Oponopono Focus: Advanced Ho'Oponopono is a powerful self-healing technique, focusing on internal issues, emotions, and personal

responsibility. It's conversational and revolves around acknowledging and transforming negative feelings about oneself.

2. Self-Responsibility: Emphasizes the concept of being 100% responsible for one's feelings and situations. Healing starts with oneself, addressing emotions, judgments, and perceptions. The process involves saying, "I am sorry, Please forgive me, Thank you, I love you."

3. Healing Frequency: Engaging in unconditional Ho'Oponopono generates a healing frequency. This involves repetitive statements, walking-talking Ho'Oponopono, and visualizing positive outcomes. The process extends beyond personal concerns to healing others and external situations.

4. Creation of Reality: Challenges the reliance on logic and past experiences, urging the abandonment of negative realistic goals. Introduces the idea that a positive, crazy goal is more beneficial than a negative, realistic one. Ho'Oponopono is presented as a tool to create a magical future.

5. Holistic Healing: Advanced Ho'Oponopono is described as healing and cleaning oneself rather than external situations. It's underscored that healing is

not about changing others but transforming one's perceptions, judgments, and emotions, contributing to a holistic approach to well-being.

4. Key Takeaways from the chapter - Elevate Your Practice: Advanced Ho'Oponopono Techniques:

1. Distinction Between Basic and Advanced Ho'Oponopono: Basic Ho'Oponopono is for others, while advanced Ho'Oponopono is a self-healing practice, addressing negative emotions within.

2. Focus on Specific Emotions: Identify and address specific negative emotions toward a person or situation. This targeted approach facilitates effective self-clearing.

3. Conversational Ho'Oponopono Technique: Engage in a conversation with yourself, using logical and conversational advanced Ho'Oponopono to heal negative emotions. This technique mirrors how healers assist others.

4. Responsibility for Personal Emotions: Acknowledge complete responsibility for the negative emotions you feel and work on clearing them. The emphasis is on self-healing, not healing others.

5. Gratitude for Negative Emotions: Express gratitude for negative emotions, recognizing that challenges contribute to personal growth. Thank yourself for the opportunities presented by these emotions.

5. Key Takeaways from the chapter - Healing Hearts, Strengthening Bonds: A Ho'Oponopono Exploration:

1. Responsibility is Key: Ho'Oponopono emphasizes taking 100% responsibility for one's feelings in relationships. This acknowledgment empowers an individual to initiate positive change.

2. Magical Resolution of Conflicts: Ho'Oponopono has a transformative impact on conflicts. By expressing forgiveness and love through specific statements, even deep-seated issues can dissolve magically.

3. Self-Healing Morning Routine: Begin your day with Ho'Oponopono for yourself. Standing in front of a mirror, say, "I'm sorry, please forgive me, thank you, I love you." Witness the magic in your self-relationship.

4. Applicability in Daily Interactions: Apply Ho'Oponopono in various life situations. Whether addressing family conflicts, seeking understanding from

a boss, or convincing colleagues, the technique is versatile and efficient.

5. Focused and Specific Practice: For optimal results, perform Ho'Oponopono for one person or purpose at a time. If dealing with multiple conflicts, maintain focus by using a photo or visualization to encompass all involved parties.

6. Key Takeaways from the chapter - The Power Of EFT With Ho'Oponopono:

1. EFT Basics: Emotional Freedom Technique (EFT), also known as tapping, involves tapping on specific energy meridian points to release emotional blockages that may cause physical and emotional issues.

2. Meridian Points and Energy Flow: EFT focuses on meridian points where energy flows in the body. By tapping on these points, one can clear energy blockages, promoting overall well-being.

3. Magical Healing: The transformative power of EFT is highlighted through a case study where a paralyzed individual, given no hope by doctors, fully recovered within three months of practicing EFT—a testament to its miraculous potential.

4. Tapping Sequence: The chapter provides a detailed tapping sequence, starting with the Karate Chop point and moving through various meridian points on the face, chest, and hands. Each point is associated with specific statements and intentions for emotional release.

5. Release Technique: The chapter introduces a personalized release technique where individuals use the statement, "Even though I am feeling this negative emotion, I love and accept myself exactly the way I am," followed by tapping on specific points while repeating the word 'release' to address specific emotions.

Note: EFT is presented as a powerful tool for emotional and physical healing, promoting the body's natural ability to self-heal by addressing energy blockages.

7. Key Takeaways from the chapter - Emotional Healing Technique:

1. NLP Basics: Neuro-linguistic programming (NLP) is introduced as a crucial technique for emotional healing. It employs communication and perceptual strategies to alter thoughts and behaviors, particularly focusing on physical pain relief.

2. Pain Transformation: NLP involves a unique process of transforming physical pain by assigning it a shape,

color, movement, size, and texture. By changing these attributes, individuals can release emotional blockages associated with pain, leading to decreased intensity.

3. Code of Emotions: NLP asserts that emotions are manufactured and changeable. The chapter explains the emotional code of "shape, color, movement, size, and texture" and how altering this code through visualization can result in emotional relief.

4. NLP with Others: The technique is shared for applying NLP to help others with pain or discomfort. By guiding them through visualizations and transformations, significant pain reduction (70-80% or even complete relief) can be achieved.

5. NLP for Emotions: NLP can be directly applied to emotional discomfort. By identifying the emotion's location, intensity, and associated details, individuals can use visualization and transformation techniques to alleviate and release emotional pain effectively. The process is described step by step for practical application.

8. Key Takeaways from the chapter - Release Technique:

1. Release Technique Introduction: The chapter introduces the Release Technique, a series of questions

aimed at releasing physical and emotional discomfort. A client's story illustrates its effectiveness in resolving marks on the body that traditional medicine couldn't address.

2. Question Sequence: The technique involves a specific sequence of questions. The first question focuses on willingness to release, followed by asking whether one should release it. The third question, crucial for physical pain, involves an immediate release, responding with "NOW."

3. Practical Example: A step-by-step example demonstrates applying the Release Technique for physical pain relief, emphasizing touching the affected area, verbalizing willingness to release, and imagining the pain dissipating with each breath.

4. Application to Various Pains: The technique is adaptable to different types of pain, demonstrated through an example addressing cold and cough symptoms. The process involves rating intensity, expressing willingness to release, and immediate release visualization.

5. Healing for Others: The Release Technique can be employed on behalf of others. By making slight modifications to the statements and using the person's

name, one can effectively perform the technique to alleviate pain or discomfort for someone else, emphasizing the interconnectedness of energy healing.

9. Key Takeaways from the chapter - Remote Healing Technique:

1. Ho'Oponopono for Parents: Take responsibility, apologize, seek forgiveness, and express love and gratitude for parents using advanced Ho'Oponopono twice daily. Experience a grounded, balanced feeling.

2. Daily Commitment: Practice advanced Ho'Oponopono consistently, morning and night, for a profound sense of balance and care.

3. Remote Healing Setup: Place a person's photo in the east, apply advanced Ho'Oponopono, and release pain through deep breaths and visualization.

4. Rethinking Pain: Challenge the notion that pain must disturb, citing an example of managing severe sciatica during workshops.

5. Emotional Control: Emphasize the power to control emotions by changing patterns, impacting overall well-being significantly.

10. Key Takeaways from the chapter - Solving Universal Problem Using Ho'oponopono Wisdom:

1. Ho'Oponopono Essence: Embrace the power of Ho'Oponopono's four humble statements: "I'm sorry, Please forgive me, Thank you, I love you." Use these positive vibrations to heal, cleanse negative energies, and attract positivity.

2. Responsibility and Healing: Ho'Oponopono begins with taking 100% responsibility for your feelings. Applying it to relationships involves self-healing, avoiding blame, and fostering positive change.

3. Addressing Negative Thoughts: Combat negative thinking by acknowledging, apologizing, and seeking forgiveness through Ho'Oponopono. Repeat the process for a set number of times, like 108, for effective results.

4. Manifesting Goals: Combine Ho'Oponopono with affirmations to manifest desires. Express gratitude, visualize the goal achieved, then follow with Ho'Oponopono for doubt-clearing. Consistency is key.

5. Healing Others: Extend Ho'Oponopono to heal ailments, even in others. Visualize health, express

responsibility, and ask for forgiveness. Consistent practice and faith in the process are crucial for positive outcomes.

Chapter 1

Soulful Cleansing: Embracing Ho'oponopono for Inner Harmony

"I love you. I'm sorry. Please forgive me. Thank you." - Dr. Ihaleakalá Hew Len, Ho'Oponopono Practitioner

What is the Ho'Oponopono technique? Many years ago, there was a doctor called Dr. Hew Len. He created a technique based on words because he realized that words have frequency. He was the mental hospital doctor of a very large hospital in a particular department called the violent department. Violent department where patients are so bad that they're killing others. They're killing themselves as well. So these patients were tied with body jackets. And their mouth is also closed because they're biting their own teeth. So these were very violent patients. Dr. Hew Len created a technique called the Ho'Oponopono technique. Using this technique, Dr. Hew Len actually cured all these violent patients in six months only. But that's not the magic part. The real magic is he cured them without medicines. And the best part, (now you're going to fall down off your chair). He not only cured them without medicine, he cured them without meeting them. Yeah!! He did not talk to them. Isn't it "pure magic"? Do you want to know what that magic is?

If you are a married woman, this technique works on your mother-in-law. My wife also uses it on my mother all the time.

I'll tell you a true story, about four or five years ago, the first time we learned Ho'Oponopono and my wife at that time, had a fight with my mother. Normal mother-in-law and Daughter in law fight. But that day, the fight was a little big. So my mother said, I will never come to your house again. Husbands generally get sandwiched between mother-in-law and daughter-in-law. So the bottom line is, my wife had learned Ho'Oponopono at that time, just knew. So she sat in one place. She thought about my mom, her mother-in-law. And she did Ho'Oponopono (the technique which I'm about to teach you.) Two days after that, mom came home with a gift. I'm not joking. And my wife did not call mom. I did not call mom. There was no physical interaction. All the interaction happened at the energy level.

So what I'm going to teach you is how to talk to people at the energy level. Convince people at the energy level, and clear energy at the energy level.

Rules of the Technique:

So there are some rules for experiencing that technique called Ho'Oponopono.

Rule number one, you have to close your eyes until the entire technique is complete. Because this is a clearing energy technique. In between, you will feel some pain. I'm warning you right now, you'll feel like crying. You'll feel like your head is aching. Sometimes you might feel like your chest is painting. It's natural. But in the middle of the surgery, pain is natural anyway. But in the middle of the surgery, you can't suddenly get up with your two kidneys in your hands and say, I want to go home now. Once the operation is started, it has to be finished.

Rule number two, when the process is going on, if you feel like crying, you will not suppress your emotions. The boys especially do this.

Rule number three, have zero body movement. As much as possible, don't move in your body language.

Steps of the Technique:

Now, before you start, bring a cloth napkin and some water. Bring a cloth napkin because when you cry, you will need it. It's a very powerful experience. First, you need to make some notes, so that we can make your mind prepared for it. Take a blank page and write down what is Ho'Oponopono? And write down the four statements: I am sorry, please forgive me, thank you, I love you. These four statements are the statements of the whole Ho'Oponopono technique. We know that all words have vibrations. These words Dr. Hew Len discovered are the most powerful frequency vibrations in the world. In fact, "I am sorry" is a very humble frequency. "I love you" is a very beautiful frequency. So he discovered that if you think of any one person and if you say these words again and again, it clears out any negative energy between you and the other person. Now this is too much theory. Let's begin the exercise.

Note: You need to do all the exercises in one sitting. And keep your eyes closed throughout the process. Your lips should be moving when you repeat the phrase.

Exercise 1: Getting prepared

First of all, follow rule number one and close your eyes. You can take a person's name. Close your eyes and place your right hand on your heart. You can play some soothing music in the background, but it also works if you want silence around you. Take a deep breath and relax.

Now repeat it loudly, your lips should be moving: *"I am sorry, please forgive me, thank you, I love you."* Say it again and again three to four times. Make sure you are not making so much movement.

Exercise 2: For Your Mother

Now Imagine your mother's face and repeat this loudly: *"I love you, mom, I'm sorry, mom. I'm really sorry. I know you did your best. I always thought you didn't love me. But I know you always love me. I'm sorry for all the hurt I gave you. I'm sorry for all the troubles I gave you. I'm really sorry, mom. Please forgive me. Thank you, mom, for always forgiving me. Thank you, mom, for always loving me. I know I did not tell you many times. But I want to tell you now, mom. I love you. I love you, mama."* Say it loudly and repeat this again.

Imagine how your mother would feel if you said this to her. Imagine she is receiving your love. Imagine her crying in happiness.

Exercise 3: For Your Father

Now, imagine your father, imagine his face. Imagine his eyes and repeat: *"I'm sorry, dad. I'm sorry for judging you. I'm sorry for not listening to you. I'm sorry for being angry with you. I know you did your best. I'm sorry for judging you. Please forgive me, dad. Thank you for giving me birth. Thank you for giving me my life. Thank you for loving me, dad. Even when I hated you many times. I love you, dad. I know I did not tell you, but I really love you. I'm really sorry, dad. Please forgive me. Thank you, dad. I love you."*

Imagine your father receiving your love. Imagine giving him a hug. How would he feel if you gave him this love? How would your father feel if you let go of all your judgment for him?

Always keep your eyes closed. No matter what you feel. Don't open your eyes.

Exercise 4: For the Person who Hurt You

Now, imagine a person in your life who hurt you the most. It may be someone in your personal life. Someone in your professional life who hurt you the most. Take that person's name and say it loudly: *"I'm sorry [that person's name]. Please forgive me. I now understand. I attracted you because of my own frequency. I'm sorry for blaming you. Please forgive me. Thank you for teaching me this lesson. Only I am responsible for my frequency. I now let you go. I now let all my hurt go away. I let go of my anger. I love you."*

And imagine you're letting the person go. You're letting the hurt go. You're letting the anger go and moving on.

Exercise 5: For Your Body

Now place both of your hands on your heart. Press it so that you can feel your heartbeat. Now repeat loudly: *"I'm sorry, dear body. I'm sorry for not taking care of you. I know I used you, overused you many times. I abused you. Please forgive me, dear body. Thank you, dear body, for keeping me healthy. I love you, dear body. I love you, my dear heart."*

Exercise 6: For Yourself

Now the last part. This time, you will be taking your own name. Keep your eyes closed. Right hand on your heart and take your own name. This time, you'll be talking to your own soul. To your own energy. So repeat it loudly: *"I'm sorry, [Your name], I know I am the one who judged you the most. I know I am the one who doubted you the most. I criticized you the most. I'm sorry for not believing in you. Please forgive me. I know I got disconnected from you. But I'm back now. I promise you. It doesn't matter who doesn't believe in you. From now on, I believe in you. It doesn't matter who doesn't love you. From now I love you. From now on, I accept you."*

Exercise 7: End Part

Now, keep both your hands across your shoulders and give yourself a hug. Right and on your left shoulder and left hand on your right shoulder. Give a warm hug. And as you give yourself a warm hug, keep your head on your shoulders, relax on yourself, and say it again: *"I'm really sorry. I'm sorry to leave you alone. Please forgive me. Thank you for still being with me. I'm back. I promise*

I'll never leave you alone." Rub your hands on your shoulders and tell yourself, "I love you." Give yourself that hug that you really deserve, and you'll realize that you were just waiting for your own love; you were just waiting for your own acceptance.

Now, for 10 seconds, relax your head on your shoulders. Give yourself that hug. Keep your eyes closed. And one last time, say it to yourself: *"I'm back. I love you."*

After doing all these parts, you can open your eyes. As you open your eyes, quickly rub your hands together a little hard and fast. Don't stop until you warm up your hands properly and now put this warmth all over your face.

This technique will make you feel relieved and super calm. It will be emotional in a beautiful way, and you will be feeling lighter after this. Imagine feeling this for 30 days. That's what the challenge is about. It's not only about feeling high, it's also about feeling calm. It's not only about creating positive frequency; it's about clearing negative energy. And both are important.

UNDERSTANDING THE BASICS: HO'OPONOPONO DEMYSTIFIED

"Ho'Oponopono is the art of taking 100% responsibility for everything in your life, because in doing so, you reclaim the power to heal and transform."

We are going to start this chapter with a story. And then we will start the Ho'Oponopono experience because this story will add even more value to the chapter.

A few years ago, there's a Commander of the Indian Air force. I am not disclosing his name. One day, he was flying as a training experience. And from his fighter plane, he had to eject a few feet below the ground. And he got so badly injured that, except for his left arm, his entire body was broken. And when I'm saying broken, it was like breaking like a stick. Like his bones were into two, three pieces. His one was leg was in very serious condition. The injury was so bad they had to operate his one particular leg and they had to reduce that by 2 cm. So when he went after the operation to the doctors in the army, in air force and talked about healing, he said, can I fly or can I go into the cockpit again? So the doctor said, you will be lucky if you can walk. And he got into low feelings and all of that. After some time, somehow he went through it. And that time his wife had purchased my book, the Law of attraction, which I did not know about. He told me when he met me for the first time that she had purchased my book law of attraction. He was lying in his house. He read that book and he tried to contact me. He sent me an email.

The moment I read him, I knew I had to talk to him. So we had a Zoom meeting and he told me about his entire story. And he said, right now the medical science says I cannot get back to service. I cannot get back to the cockpit. I want to fly again. It's my passion. I want to serve my country once again. And can you help me? I said 'yes.' He was very surprised. Because he thought I would say it's not possible enough. And I still remember what I told him that day. I said, a crazy goal, a positive crazy goal, is much better than a negative realistic goal. So maybe it is realistic that you cannot fly again. And maybe it's true, right? And maybe it's crazy to believe that you can fly again. But at least what is better, a positive crazy goal is better than a negative realistic goal. So I agreed to work with him with the only condition that he will meet me every day on Zoom live. And for the next one month, we worked with him every single day. For three and a half years, almost every day, he's never missed a session. And he kept working and working and recently he sent me a message.

That miracle has happened, which we had imagined. And for that one month when we worked with each other, we used to keep visualizing that he's flying in a plane where I would download videos from YouTube where he would have these 3d virtual views of a cockpit. And the plane is flying with the same sound and everything. And I would make him visualize that he's taking turns now. Because he was a pilot. It was very easy for him to remember that he's taking off, he's going. So all those videos when I played for him, it was very realistic for him. But his legs couldn't move. I said to him that the mind can make the leg move, but you have to train the mind to make the leg move. Believe it or not, with his commitment, the man was such that they found the right doctor in the air force. They surgically, literally move,cut his leg, put a piece of bone inside, covered it up with a structure which is a kind of bracket. And inside that, the bone grew back by a centimeter. And he was once again after three years of hard work, became fit and qualified for the exam of a pilot once more. He messaged me his picture flying a fighter plane and said: "I just finished my first flight and the picture is here". He finished his first flight. And he's now back in the Airforce. And the best part, he's serving fully fledged, and he's promoted. So earlier he was just a commander. Now he's a group captain.

Now let's learn about how we can use this feeling to understand what is the magical world that we are into right now. Because we are definitely not in the world of logic. We are in the world of Magic. But to be in that world of magic, the number one rule that you have to follow is- don't use logic. Why? Because logic is based on the experience.

If everybody will work on past experience, then how would you create the future? To create the future, you have to ignore the past. You have to forget what the past says about what is possible and what is not possible.

And to do that, one of the best mediums in life, one of the best tools in life that we have learned, is called Ho'Oponopono. And there's a difference between basic Ho'Oponopono and advanced Ho'Oponopono.

Let's understand basic Ho'Oponopono first. Basic Ho'Oponopono is a simple repetition of four statements. The basic Ho'Oponopono is focused on outside people, outside situations, outside incidents and anything outside. Anything outside is for basic Ho'Oponopono. We don't do basic Ho'Oponopono for ourselves; the advanced Ho'Oponopono is for ourselves.

If you want to do Ho'Oponopono for your father, you need to do basic Ho'Oponopono. If you're doing Ho'Oponopono to get a job, that's basic Ho'Oponopono. Something is not working in your house and you're doing basic Ho'Oponopono. So whenever you're doing Ho'Oponopono for something outside you, it is always basic Ho'Oponopono.

How does it work? It is very simple. You need to do this 108 times twice in a day and you need to do unconditional practice. What is unconditional practice? Most people do Ho'Oponopono for a particular condition, for a particular thing, for a particular person.

But we don't do it only for a purpose, we do it unconditionally. Twice in a day, 108 times.

You should do the unconditional Ho'Oponopono 108 times, twice a day because you need to start realizing the power of basic Ho'Oponopono. There are three steps you should follow every day. First and second is morning and evening Ho'Oponopono, 108 times and third step is walking-talking Ho'Oponopono. What do we do about this? Walking-talking Ho'Oponopono is Ho'Oponopono. You can do anytime doesn't matter where you are and what you are doing. You're having some conversation with your friend and suddenly your friend feels bad about something. Immediately start doing walking-talking Ho'Oponopono for your friend. You're going for a movie, there's a long queue you do walking-talking Ho'Oponopono for the queue so that you've reached on time. If you see any person feeling any trouble in his/her life, you will immediately do walking-talking Ho'Oponopono for them.

So let's do some walking-talking right now. Think of somebody or some situation in your life which requires a little healing. Do Ho'Oponopono for that person or that situation eleven times right now while you are reading this book. Say: "I'm sorry, Please forgive me, Thank you, I love you. Do this four to five times. The moment you've done this, you've generated something around you. Can you make a guess? What have you generated? The frequency of Ho'Oponopono. And that is a healing frequency in itself. So walking-talking Ho'Oponopono has to be done the whole day. The moment there is a negative situation or a person, you can do instant healing with walking-talking Ho'Oponopono.

CHAPTER 3

BEYOND BASICS: ADVANCED HO'OPONOPONO MASTERY

"Forgiveness is the key to action and freedom." - Morrnah Nalamaku Simeona, Creator of Self-Identity through Ho'Oponopono

The basic Ho'Oponopono is always done outside and advanced Ho'Oponopono is done inside, which means we never do advanced Ho'Oponopono for somebody else. We may teach somebody to do advanced Ho'Oponopono for themselves, but you are not doing advanced Ho'Oponopono for them. You're always doing Ho'Oponopono for yourself. Advance Ho'Oponopono is also called conversational Ho'Oponopono. Basic Ho'Oponopono is like repetition again and again, but advanced Ho'Oponopono is different. There are two rules: Rule number one, we are only doing it for ourselves. So whenever you're doing advanced hope no, first you have to check step number one. What specific emotion or person are you doing advanced Ho'Oponopono for? We can do it for TSP (things, situations, and people). Whenever you're doing advanced Ho'Oponopono.

Step one is to write down specifically that you are doing Ho'Oponopono for a thing or situation or person.

Step two; you need to be sure about what negative emotion you have about either this thing, this situation, or this person?

Advanced Ho'Oponopono basically means heal and clean. It is about your feelings about things, situations, and people. For example, if you are worried about somebody, you don't need to heal them first. You need to heal your worry that you feel for them first. Now you would say, but Sooraj, isn't it natural that I'm worried about my father? No, it's not natural, it is learned. Trees are green, that's natural. Water removes your thirst, that's natural. Food gives you energy, that's natural. Every person in the world has to worry for their father. Is that natural? No. God has not made us like that. Universe has not made us like that. Nature already exists. The rest we have created by ourselves. So we have learned to worry about people. It's not natural. So when you're worried about someone, you don't want to heal them. You want to heal your worries for them. And that is called healing and cleaning our energy.

When Dr. Hew Len did this exercise with his mental patients, do you think he was really healing and cleaning? He was not healing and cleaning them. He was healing and cleaning how he was feeling about them. For example, he would go to the Hospital, he would open the report of one patient. And he would read about a person saying he was a criminal, and he killed somebody. Now, the moment you read the person has killed somebody, what happens? Judgment appears. You start feeling bad for the person. It's normal. The moment that happens, Dr. Hew Len said, start healing and cleaning how you are feeling about that person and you will heal that person.

Let me explain the logic behind it. At the energy level, we are all one. I am energy and you are also energy. If I start worrying about your health, your bad health and my worries are at the same frequency. Lock and key have the same frequency. Your health problem and my worry problem have the same frequency.

You must have never heard this before: *Because I have the capacity to worry, I manifest people who have problems.* Because I have the capacity to worry. I literally manifest problems in people so I can worry about them. Sometimes you're literally making people sick so that you can worry. It's not possible otherwise. The existence of worry requires existence of a problem (a health problem or a relationship problem or a career problem or a financial problem). And because I have the capacity to worry, I'm creating that problem in my life. The more you feel bad about politics in the country, guess what will happen in the country? More politics.

Does the universe have the capacity to create such big things? Yes. Or course. And because you have the capacity to make somebody sick, you also have the capacity to make somebody healed. You have the capacity to make somebody struggle in their life. So if you keep worrying about your younger brother or sister. They will struggle more. If you are able to heal your capacity of worry, their problem will disappear. Their struggle has to disappear.

Let's have another example: in our society there are certain girls who are eligible for marriage. They look good and have very good character and also make money. There is not a single flaw in them, but still they are not getting married. The biggest reason why that girl doesn't get married is because of the worry of the parents. Her parents are so much worried about her marriage and they are worried how she will survive after marriage. And because of that, her parents keep finding faults with every boy that comes in her life. The marriage of that girl will keep getting delayed and delayed. In some cases I have seen some girls getting divorce later.

If you don't heal your capacity to worry, you will create problems in life. The more you worry about somebody, the more you are cursing that person. So the moment you see a problem in someone's life, the first person you will heal is always you, yourself. If you feel that person needs the healing, you're judging them, which means you require healing first. That thought, that feeling, requires healing first. If you're worried about someone, you require healing first.

But how do we do this healing? We use a technique called advanced Ho'Oponopono, which I discovered over a period of years. You will not find this in any book in the world. Because this is something I created over a period of years. In fact, even if you go and do Joe Vitale's or Dr. Hew Len's video of Ho'Oponopono you will not find this technique there. Also, because it's something that I've created over a period of conversational Ho'Oponopono. The technique is very simple. Let's see the script first, then I'll explain the technique, how it works.

The step one of the scripts is- *"I am 100% responsible for the way I feel."* That always is the first line. Then you will start saying: "I am sorry (Multiple reasons). Please forgive me (Multiple reasons). Thank you (Multiple reasons). I love you (Multiple reasons). These reasons have to be written down in your notepad and should be spontaneous and honest. When you're doing conversational Ho'Oponopono, it is better to do it with music.

Let's understand with an example: I am telling you the story of my friend. He was looking for trouble so I asked him what the problem was. He said: "I'm out of my job. And after that I met with an accident while I was in Hyderabad. I had two surgeries on my left leg. And then I'm also diagnosed with intestinal TB, which is also in progress." Now imagine yourself in his situation and do Ho'Oponopono for this.

Ho'Oponopono Technique:

First of all, place your hands on your heart and take a deep breath. You can start music in the background. In advance Ho'Oponopono you don't need to close your eyes. You can keep your eyes open. So it's like having a conversation. Say:

"I take 100% responsibility for the way I feel and for all these situations that I have attracted and created. All my dear problems. I'm sorry for hating you. I'm sorry for feeling sad for you. Because the fact is I created you. How can I hate you when I have created you? Please forgive me for not realizing all the benefits you give me. I know I'm enjoying the benefits, but I am not acknowledging it. Please forgive me for that. Please forgive me for thinking you should have not come into my life. The fact is that you did not come. I literally gave you birth. I created you. And then I disowned you as if you are baggage. The fact is that I gave birth to you. So thank you for being in my life. Thank you for teaching me all the lessons. Thank you for giving me this amazing experience. I would have never started practicing the Ho'Oponopono without these problems; I don't have a job. Thank you for that. I got the time to practice and master this magic. Thank you for being in my life. Thank you for all the benefits that I experience consciously or unconsciously. So many people love me because of this and sympathize with me. And make me comfortable and give me extra attention. I give myself extra attention all because of these problems. So thank you for all these benefits. Dear problems, I love you,

I really love you and I'm really sorry for hating you, I'm really sorry for hating you."

Now think of your job not being there. And all the time that you spent without a job, think that time is like a human being you're talking to and say:

<u>*"I'm sorry, sorry for hating you. I love you. I love spending that time with you. Anyways, when I die I won't be taking my job with me. But I'll definitely take my feelings with me. So thank you so, thank you for the wisdom. For the wisdom to master my feelings. The fact is I would have never even tried to master my feelings without these problems. So thank you and I love you."*</u>

You must be feeling very light. Think about your job not being there. You will feel great. Think about your TB. You will find it's gone. Now you can do this for your problem and you will find them going away from you.

Let's take one more example here: there was a lady whose son was autistic. There was so much worry between her and her husband and their relationship was breaking down because of her son. Her husband wanted her to take care of the boy totally. So it was very important that her son was healed. So we are not going to heal her son with the Ho'Oponopono, whom are we going to heal? Her. Because the problem is not about her son.

The problem is about how her husband treats her and how she feels about her son. So we need to first heal her, not her son.

So let's begin. Place your hands on your heart. Turn on some music. And say:

"I take 100% responsibility for the way I am feeling. For the way I am feeling in this whole situation. I take 100% responsibility for creating this situation. The fact is, my son just has a problem which is actually not troubling him so much. It's me who's getting troubled. And I am creating this troubling feeling. So I am responsible for this feeling. My husband thinks I have to take care of my son all the time. I'm responsible for that. I'm sorry for creating this for myself. I didn't create my son's autism, but I definitely created how I feel about him. So I am sorry for feeling so much pity for him. I am sorry for the anger and frustration I feel. Please forgive me for believing my husband is responsible for the way I feel. Please forgive me for believing that if my son is healed, all my problems will be solved. I know that's not true. Because even if my son is healed, I will find another reason to worry. Feeling like a victim feeling like a victim has been my habit for many years before even my son came into my life. I'm used to feeling like a victim. So thank you, my dear son, for making me realize to stop giving myself all that bullshit. Thank you for reminding me. I

don't prioritize myself. My husband is not the problem. I feel guilty if I prioritize myself. If I prioritize myself. Fact is, more than my husband, I should sacrifice for my son. So I don't give any time to myself. But because I can't hate myself, I started blaming my husband. But the fact is that I created this victim. So thank you, my dear husband, for pushing me to say no. Because the fact is how will I have the opportunity to say no if he doesn't expect too much from me? My real test is not how much he prioritizes me, but how much I prioritize myself. Thank you, my dear husband, for ignoring me so that someone else can find me. I'll find myself. I love you, my dear son, with your autism. You can be like this all your life. I give you the freedom to be yourself. I created you this way. You seem to love yourself this way. So now I started to love you. If you have autism, you have the freedom to have that so that now I can have the freedom to find time for myself. So I can create time for myself. I love you, dear husband."

This is how you can make affirmations for your problems and can heal yourself.

I hope you are now 100% clear that Advanced Ho'Oponopono is for healing and cleaning yourself. So the moment you see a problem in life as an advanced magician, as Ho'Oponopono healers. The first person you will heal is who? Always yourself.

Quick Review of the process:

Now, think of a situation, thing, or a person, and write down all the negative feelings that you feel about it. For example, sadness, anger, guilt, frustration, anything you have just written it down. We do not heal that thing outside. We are healing the way we are feeling about that thing, situation, and person. How do we do that? Always take one feeling at a time. Once you've taken that feeling, then you ask yourself the level of feeling at the level of one to ten. One is low and ten is high. Now you start saying advanced Ho'Oponopono for yourself. If your problem is 'anger' you say like this: "I am 100% responsible for this situation that is making me angry, (and now you create multiple reasons why you're saying sorry), after this you start saying, thank you, sorry, please forgive me (with multiple reasons). You keep doing this, and then in the end, you ask yourself, what is the level of the anger now? This time, the rating will be closer to zero. Now you do one more round and check for the rating again. We need to repeat the same process until the rating reaches zero. You don't stop before that.

You can directly take an entire situation, and a story, and you dissolve that story completely. And because you dissolve that story, suddenly all the emotions with that have gone. All the beliefs have gone; everything has just gone, disappeared.

Let's take an example again: this time we will be healing a person who has the feeling of lacking money. So let's work on that. First of all, this person needs to place his hands on his heart and put on some music. Take a deep breath and say: *"I'm 100% responsible for the way I feel about money. For the way I feel about you. Sometimes I feel it is there, sometimes I feel it is not there. I'm sorry for ignoring all those beautiful moments where I always had enough money for whatever I needed. I'm really sorry for creating this lack of money feeling. I created this feeling. Please forgive me for judging it. Now I realize actually what is so wrong about having less money. Everything is taken care of, so please forgive me. Please forgive me for judging this feeling. I hate this idea of lack of money. Thank you for giving me the ability to create abundance. Instead of hating it, I love this lack. I love less money also and more money as well. I love 'lack' and 'abundance' as well. So I love you, dear Money. Whether you come in lack or in abundance, you're always welcome. You're welcome whether you come in crores, thousands or just in hundreds. I love you the way you are."* Take a deep breath!

Now this person will check the level of intensity on the scale of one to ten. What was the feeling of lack of money earlier? And what is it now? When I asked this person, he replied: Earlier it was almost eight and after the first round it was two.

Now it's time to heal you. The first thing I want you to heal is the feeling that someone else needs to heal you. And that someone else can be anyone like your friend, family member or a random person on the street you feel bad for. After you can pick up your other feelings only by and start healing yourself with Ho'Oponopono.

'Should' and 'Must' things:

There are two kinds of things in life: Should things and Must things. A 'should' is something good to have and a 'must' is that you must have. What is juice? It is a 'should' thing. What is water? It's a must. Human beings are so powerful, once we make something a must, we make it happen, and then we never look back. The problem is we don't call it a must. 90% of the goals of human beings are not achieved because we think our goals are 'should' things. That's why we don't achieve our goals, because we call them this should happen.

Do you remember the story of that commander I discussed earlier in the book? He took three years to heal and to go back to being a pilot. In the first year, he could have given up. Second year, he could have given up. Third year, he could have given up. The reason he's successful at his goal, because he believed that 'once a pilot, always a pilot'. He said, I'm a pilot and I'm going back. I don't know how I'm going back. And for him, it was not a 'should' thing; he believed he must have to be a pilot again. He's not going to look back.

When you become a healer, you cannot make it a 'should'. It has to be a 'must'. You can't go back to being a normal person anymore. You're a magical healer. So you can heal your life, so you can heal other's lives and inspire your students to heal their lives. And that is why your responsibility is to never stop healing, never stop learning.

CHAPTER 4

ELEVATE YOUR PRACTICE: ADVANCED HO'OPONOPONO TECHNIQUES

"Cleaning is not just erasing memories but clearing the path for inspiration to enter." - Dr. Ihaleakalá Hew Len

This lesson is all about **Advanced Ho'Oponopono.**

Now the first question comes into our mind is that- what is the difference between basic Ho'Oponopono

And advanced Ho'Oponopono? Let's understand that first. Basic Ho'Oponopono is what we learn from YouTube and the internet which is simply thinking of a particular person, or thinking of yourself, or maybe thinking of your exams, or thinking of any person in the world or any situation in the world or thinking of your goal and simply saying affirmations.

You may have done the basic Ho'Oponopono, and you must be surprised by its results. Now imagine if basic Ho'Oponopono has already given you amazing results, how amazing the advance Ho'Oponopono will be. The first thing to understand is that basic Ho'Oponopono is for other people and advanced is for yourself.

Say this like an affirmation: "basic Ho'Oponopono is for other people and advanced Ho'Oponopono is for me.

Now what do I mean by that? What is the purpose of Ho'Oponopono? The purpose of Ho'Oponopono is for clearing negative energy. So whenever we're doing basic Ho'Oponopono, we're clearing negative energy from inside or outside for other people. But when we're doing advanced Ho'Oponopono, we're not clearing for other people, we're clearing for ourselves. You do it for the emotions you feel for other people. Let's take an example.

Think about the person with whom you get upset with very quickly. It can be anybody, your brother, mother, sister, father, colleague, boss, subordinate. It can be somebody from the past. He/she is the person with whom you're a little bit disturbed.

The way to use advanced Ho'Oponopono is to always start with thinking about one situation or one specific person. Either one situation or one person. You can take a notepad and write instead of thinking. Writing gives better results. And then you write down your emotions with that person. Negative emotions you feel towards that situation or towards that person.

What are the emotions you feel towards these people? Is it anger? Is it frustration? Is it helplessness? Write down all those emotions. Now, some of those emotions may not be just one emotion. It may be multiple emotions. All these emotions you are thinking or writing about have a negative frequency. The emotions are inside you because you are feeling these emotions. So where is the frequency right now? Inside you. So who do we need to clean? Ourselves. So, advanced in Ho'Oponopono, Dr. Hew Len says, is never about clearing other people's energy, it's about clearing our energy.

Now, how do we do that? First, we always take a specific situation or a specific person. We've already done that.

Second, we write down what specific negative emotions we are experiencing towards the situation or towards the person? We've also done that.

The third step is where we start practicing advanced Ho'Oponopono. All we need to do is:

Put your hand on your heart and repeat, you will always start with the statement which is "I take 100% responsibility for all the negative emotions I feel towards this situation or towards this person." Immediately after saying that, we take one emotion and we start clearing that emotion within us by saying logical advanced Ho'Oponopono. It's also called conversational advanced Ho'Oponopono. By this technique, healers heal others. What you need to do here is have a conversation with the person whom you're healing in advanced Ho'Oponopono. Whom are you healing? Always yourself. So whom are you going to have this conversation with? Yourself. But how do you have a conversation?

If I tell you to give a public speaking speech, you might have to write a script. But if you're having a conversation with your best friend, do you write a script down? No, it's a conversation and we don't need a script for that. So the way to do it is to have a session with yourself in the Ho'Oponopono format. For example, I had a client, and

I was having a session with her. I asked her to tell me the emotion that she's dealing with.

She said: *"So the emotion I have currently is for a friend, it's a lot of trust issues. I feel very angry. I mean, the way he has after knowing some of my secrets, the way he has behaved with me or made fun of me or the situation, it made me feel very bad. I tried to talk to him, but he was not understanding and I felt very bad about the entire situation."*

I asked her: did he make fun of you?

She said: yes.

I asked: He didn't talk to you properly?

She said: *"No, he is very disrespectful, I respect him but he don't, I am feeling disrespectful and very angry, I tried to talk but it didn't work, and now I have stopped talking but it is giving me a lot of uncomforted feeling because I used to respect him as an elder brother."*

I hope my readers got the situation in this case. Now just replace yourself with her. Now we're going to use the conversational Ho'Oponopono exercise to heal her.

So the first emotion she described was disrespect. We will write down this specific emotion to start with. We can't take all emotions at the same time. We've chosen disrespect in this case. At first we will check the intensity of this negative emotion on a level of one to ten. Eight would be low and ten would be very high. When I asked her, she said 'eight'.

Now we need the duration for which you are dealing with this emotion.

I asked: You've been dealing with this emotion for how long now?

She said: Almost a month.

And for a month, you've never been able to reduce this from eight to zero or eight to three?

She replied: Whenever I think it bothers me a lot, actually, it was more than eight.

So I'll show you how you will think about him, and yet the emotion will go down. But for that, you have to clean yourself. You have to heal yourself. You have to clear your own negative emotions of feeling disrespectful.

Try to feel positive first and place your hands on your heart. (We are going to use a particular emotion which is disrespect, but you can do this for the negative emotion that you want to clear.) Circulate your hand over your heart like you're cleaning a whiteboard and repeat: *"I take 100% responsibility for feeling disrespectful and I understand this is my frequency, this is my emotional pattern, when I look in my past, I can remember many instances where I have experienced the same emotion for different reasons. So the fact is, only I am responsible for feeling disrespectful. This is my emotional habit and I will change it forever."*

Feel your past and imagine you are healing from that. Now repeat: "I'm really sorry for putting all this blame on me. I attracted this situation because I have a habit of feeling disrespectful because this is my frequency, because this is my emotional habit. I realize that now and I'm really sorry for blaming myself. Please forgive me for holding on to this emotion."

Now repeat the third phrase: "I have disrespected myself and hated myself so much because I thought I am different from me but now I know we both are one. So I love me, and I will love me the way I love myself. I forgive myself because there are so many times I have disrespected myself. I can forgive myself.

Now keep your eyes closed and just think of that person, think of that situation. Relax! Now just check how you're feeling. So you can open your eyes. Now you must be feeling great. If you think you need to do this one more time, go for it and repeat everything again.

Are you feeling overly charged? Yin or Yang? Good or bad? Right or wrong? No, it's just balance right now. This is the power of simply allowing yourself to heal one person. Who's that? Yourself. Now, after this exercise, rate yourself from 1 to 10 again. This was your first round of advanced Ho'Oponopono and you can see the significant decrease in the rating. This is called healing yourself or cleaning yourself in advanced Ho'Oponopono. We are never ever, ever cleaning anybody else. We are only cleaning ourselves.

If you are upset with your mother-in-law, you will be doing healing for whom in advance Ho'Oponopono? For yourself. All the emotions that you feel for your mother-in-law. Now, the way you're supposed to do it is you will write down first each emotion and write down the intensity of that emotion. And then you will keep doing advanced Ho'Oponopono, which means conversational Ho'Oponopono with yourself until that number goes down to zero. You have to keep repeating this until the number goes down to zero. Then you will take the second emotion you feel for that person. As in the above-mentioned lady had 'anger' as her second feeling of emotion against that man. So you also have to take all emotions for the same person and clear them out one by one until the number goes to zero.

This entire exercise will take 10 to 15 minutes, depending on how many emotions are there?

You may be thinking that 10 to 15 minutes are too long, but imagine how long you've been stuck with these emotions. Even 20 minutes is nothing in front of that long duration. Isn't it worth investing 15 minutes in one go to let go of this emotion forever? So please do it.

Now the question that comes in your mind is that in the statement above, why am I thanking myself for creating the negative emotion? Because you have become who you have become, not because of your positive emotions, but because of the challenges your negative emotions gave you. The negative emotions also serve you. So you have to thank yourself for that emotion.

Now we're going to do one more round. But this time, we're going to take something very deadly. Something which you are scared of healing. I want you to do the same activity one more time. But take a situation or a person whom you're scared of and start healing yourself. We are doing this because we are not basic Ho'Oponopono; we are advanced Ho'Oponopono practitioners. Take your second hand and give yourself a high five and say, I am an advanced Ho'Oponopono practitioner. Now, get ready. I'm going to tell you what advanced people do when they see someone getting hurt.

And if you are feeling bad for them being hurt, whom do you have to Ho'Oponopono for feeling hurt? If God feels hurt, will you feel bad for God? No. Because you know, God can take care of God. Because you trust in God. So when you feel bad for others not taking care of themselves, what energy are you passing them? Negative energy. So you don't have to heal them in advance. You have to heal whom? Yourself. So that's why I repeat in advance Ho'Oponopono that we never heal other people. If there's a beggar going on the road, and if you're feeling bad about the beggar, whom are you going to heal? Yourself.

In advance Ho'Oponopono, the rule is very simple. We are taking responsibility for everything we are feeling and we are creating. We are not healing the other person; we are healing ourselves.

So get yourself ready to take something deadly. Place your right hand on your heart and say the statement: "I am hundred percent responsible for the way I feel...." Give yourself a logical reason for feeling this, give yourself a reason to say sorry, give yourself a reason to forgive, give yourself a reason to thank, give yourself a reason to love. Keep your eyes closed, take a deep breath. Relax your energy. And just check how you're feeling. Usually, people get so emotional during the session. That's the point where the feelings are getting lighter through your tears. You must be feeling very relaxed, very calm because it was all hidden deep inside you.

Your questions will not answer anything. Your practice will answer everything.

HEALING HEARTS, STRENGTHENING BONDS: A HO'OPONOPONO EXPLORATION

*"By taking responsibility, we
uncover the peace within us and
contribute to the peace of the world."
- Morrnah Nalamaku Simeona*

Let's learn how to use Ho'Oponopono for relationships in this chapter. In this chapter, we are going to talk about how we use the most powerful technique of the law of attraction, which is Ho'Oponopono, to improve our relationships.

Whenever you are doing Ho'Oponopono for somebody else, the first statement you must always say is "I take 100% responsibility for my feelings." The moment you say that, you're saying that you have the ultimate power to take responsibility for your relationships. But if you believe that the other person has to change, the other person has to do something, the other person has to behave in a certain way for your relationship to improve, and then Ho'Oponopono doesn't work. So the first statement always has to start with responsibility. "I take 100% responsibility to improve this relationship. I take 100% responsibility for whatever is going on in my relationship right now." Then, after that simple technique, take that person's name and say: "I am sorry, please forgive me. Thank you. I love you for that person in your mind or loudly, about 108 times." If the relationship is at a very critical stage, then you can say Ho'Oponopono 108 times for them twice a day." But if it's at a critical stage, let's say you've had a little argument with someone, think of that person and say the Ho'Oponopono: "I'm sorry, please forgive me. Thank you. I love you." Say these four statements about eleven times and then just leave it.

What happens when you say these statements to the other person? The negativity between you and the other person gets cleaned up. Let me give you an example of my real life. The first time we discovered this technique was when my wife was not getting along with my mom. It was a typical mother-in-law, daughter-in-law problem. And when she was not getting along, my mentor taught my wife Ho'Oponopono. And all she did was she took my mom's name, and she said: "I'm sorry mom. Please forgive me mom. Thank you mom for everything. I love you mom." And that's it! She did this about eleven times. The fight was so critical at that time that mom had actually said that she'll never come back to my house again. Next day after my wife does this Ho'Oponopono, you won't believe that my mom came home with a gift saying beta, whatever happened, forget it and let's move on. This is actually a true story and normally these kinds of conflicts don't dissolve very easily. But the reason this conflict dissolved was not because of logic, but because of magic. Ho'Oponopono is really magical.

Now let me show you where you can use Ho'Oponopono in your relationships. When you get up in the morning, the first person whom you have a relationship with is yourself. So first of all, you should do Ho'Oponopono for yourself. In the morning, go to the mirror, when you're brushing your teeth, just look at yourself and say: "hey [your name], I'm sorry. Please forgive me. Thank you. I love you." Do it for a couple of days and see the magic that you have in your own relationship with yourself. After you do Ho'Oponopono for yourself, you can do this for anybody whom you deal with in the family, while you're talking to them. If you had an argument with someone, mentally think about that person and say: "I'm sorry, please forgive me. Thank you. I love you." Suddenly, the conflict will disappear.

You are on the way to the office and on the way you're thinking about whether your boss will listen to you, whether your boss will not listen to you. Simply take your boss's name and say, "I'm sorry, please forgive me. Thank you. I love you."

After you have reached the office and you're having a meeting, you want your other colleagues to be convinced by the presentation that you're giving. Take their name and say: "I'm sorry, please forgive me. Thank you. I love you." The application of Ho'Oponopono is at so many places. The point is, think about that person and say: "I'm sorry, please forgive me. Thank you. I love you." And then see the magic that happens in just two to five minutes, maximum.

You may be getting confused about doing Ho'Oponopono for multiple purposes in a single go. Always do Ho'Oponopono at one time for one thing. You can do it for multiple things, but then in that case, don't take any name. You can simply say: "I'm sorry, please forgive me. Thank you. I love you." But if you want to do Ho'Oponopono for specific things, don't combine all those things and do it in one go. One Ho'Oponopono for one person at a time gives better results.

If you are having arguments with two or three persons are a time, like if you are having arguments with your wife and your mother at the same time, try to have one single photo where both persons are together. And then look at both of them and say: "I'm sorry. Please forgive me. Thank you. I love you 108 times twice a day."

If you want to get married, you can say these affirmations: "I'm already happily married and I'm very happy with my new life partner" You can even add: "I went to this particular place for my honeymoon. We have come back and we are having a very happy married life."

How to pray for a lady whose divorce is in court to help her get back to her husband? You can take their photograph as a couple. Look at both of them together and say these affirmations: "thank you, universe. Both these people are now very happy living with each other once again. Loving each other once again."

What affirmations can you say for good earnings? You can say: "whatever I am feeling about lack of earning, I take responsibility for that. I am sorry. Please forgive me. Thank you. I love you." Clean up this emotion of whatever negative you're feeling with fewer earnings. And you start saying "I have amazing earnings. Now I'm making 50% more money compared to my last month for any negative feeling that was stopping me from earning this. I'm sorry. Please forgive me. Thank you. I love you."

You can make statements of every condition, and for any person. So start doing Ho'Oponopono from today and see the results.

MAY I ASK YOU FOR A SMALL FAVOR?

I want to express my sincere gratitude for choosing to invest your time in reading this book. Your decision to explore this work among countless others means a lot to me.

I hope that within these pages, you've discovered actionable insights that can enhance your daily life. Your journey doesn't have to end here, though.

May I kindly request an additional 30 seconds of your valuable time?

Sharing your thoughts about the book through a review would be immensely appreciated. Your review serves as a beacon, guiding other readers to take a chance on my books. It's a small gesture that carries significant weight in the world of authors.

To submit your review effortlessly, please **Scan** the **QR Code** below. It will take you directly to the book's review page:

"The Alchemy of Healing" or "Global Link"

Alternatively, you can also find the "**Reviews Section**" of this book's page on Amazon.

Your review will require just a minute of your time but will make a monumental difference in helping me connect with a broader audience and I eagerly look forward to reading your review.

Once again, thank you for your unwavering support of my work.

CHAPTER 6

THE POWER OF EFT WITH HO'OPONOPONO

When you say 'I'm sorry,' you are taking responsibility. You are not saying you are sorry for what you did, but you are saying you are sorry for what you are feeling." – Morrnah Nalamaku Simeona

What is EFT?

Emotional Freedom Technique (EFT) is a therapy that involves tapping on the body's energy meridians to release emotional blockages. EFT is also known as tapping, and it involves tapping on different parts of the face and chest.

EFT works because there are certain meridian points in our body. These meridian points are like channels. For example, the area where your index finger joins your palm. There is a connection, there is a channel. If somebody hits over here, the part on the top and the part at the bottom, both will get affected. Because this is the main thing connecting to both parts. Just like this, there are certain meridian points from where energy flows. And if the energy is blocked in those particular energy blocks or those energy meridian points, it starts creating health problems within your body. Physical problems, emotional problems start happening.

All our emotions are made up of energy. And energy has frequency. So if you tap at a particular point in your body, which is known as the meridian points, by tapping on those points, you're releasing the energy and the frequency of that energy in those particular points.

For example, assume there is water not coming in the tap of your house. And as per the society, the pipeline is working, but the water is not coming in the tap of your house. So many times the plumber will come and he'll hammer on the pipe. When he hammers, many times the dirt which is inside the taps releases. And as a result of that, the water starts flowing again. You may have had this experience. Sometimes you just have to clear up blockages. Just like that, we have energy blockages in our body. EFT gives you the ability to release energy blocks in your body from certain meridian points.

How to do EFT?

First part is called the Karate Chop point, also called KC. The Karate Chop point (abbreviated KC) is located at the center of the fleshy part of the outside of your hand (either hand) between the top of the wrist and the base of the baby finger. The karate chop point is the first point and the last point, which means you start with the karate chop, you end with the karate chop. Many people do the entire EFT only with this, nothing else. When we do the release technique, we'll simply do this. That whatever is causing this pain, physically or emotionally, unconsciously or unconsciously, am I willing to release it? Yes. And then you take a deep breath. So only doing this one point can create amazing results for you.

The biggest reason why I got attracted to EFT was a case study, which I read about by the founder of EFT. The case study was about the person who came to his workshop. He was completely paralyzed, and he was in a wheelchair, and doctors had told him that he will never walk for the rest of his life. This man got completely cured of paralysis in three months using EFT. For me, this is like beyond magic, it's like a miracle. And then I started doing more and more research on it and realized that the power of EFT is just amazing.

In this chapter, we will learn the power of how to do it and where to do it. So, first is the karate chop point. Then take your first two fingers together and put them on the beginning of your eyebrows and tap here. When you're tapping, be careful. You're not supposed to hurt yourself. Make sure you don't have very sharp nails when you are tapping. Or if you have very sharp nails, tap it this way that you're not hurting. Then start tapping under your eyeballs and on the top of your head, at the center of your head, tap with both your hands and both your fingers. Now, tap on upper lips and after this on lower lips. And now tap on the point where your collarbone meets sternum. After this, tap under your underarms one by one. After this, tap the side of your fingers and thumb just below the nail (the point where the skin and the nail attach together). Start with your thumb. After you tap the thumb, move to the first finger, the second one, the third one, the fourth one. This way, you tap all four fingers. We started with a karate chop point and we will end with a karate chop point.

The founder of the EFT technique gave an amazing technique. Write the statement on your notepad: "Even though I am feeling this negative emotion, I love and accept myself exactly the way I Am." say this twice or thrice. The reason you need to say this statement particularly is whenever we have any negative emotion going on, who is the first person we are upset with? Ourselves. And that is why many times we say in anger, *why do I do this with myself?* So you need to first let go of that anger. And you need to say the opposite of anger, which is love and acceptance. The best way to heal is not to pour more hurt on hurt, but to add more medicine on hurt. So the love and acceptance is the best medicine for all kinds of hurts in life.

So this is how we start. Tap your karate chop point and repeat this loudly: Even though I am feeling this negative emotion, I love and accept myself exactly the way I am. Now, when you're saying this negative emotion, when you do the exercise, you're going to use the same emotion that you're working on. For example, even though I am feeling frustrated, I love and accept myself exactly the way I am. Even though I'm feeling helpless, I love and accept myself the way I am. So you will say this three times for the same emotion. And then you will tap on all the points while saying the word 'release' after that.

Now, this is not something you'll find in any EFT manual. It's something I've discovered over a period of time. The subconscious mind works very powerfully when you use the word 'release.'

Now, similarly, you keep going through all the points while saying the same word. For example, frustration 'release', all my frustration 'release'. Any frustration I have, 'release'. You can see a little bit of variation of that, but basically you're saying frustration release if you're using it for sadness, same thing: all my sadness, 'Release.' If you're using it for helplessness, say the same thing- all my helplessness, 'Release'. If you're feeling not good enough, then you're going to say this feeling of not good enough- 'Release'.

Think about the emotion you want to clear. The emotion can be **irritation, anger, sadness, upset; frustration, self doubt, hatred, jealousy, feeling low, feeling neglected, feeling ignored, desperation** etc. give this emotion a rating on the scale of one to ten. Ten means intensity of emotion is very high and one means very low. Turn on some music and start practicing the EFT technique. In this technique, you don't need to necessarily keep your eyes open. In fact, it's good to keep the eyes open because then you know where you're tapping. Keep tapping according to the sequence and say: "even though I'm [angry] with myself, I love and accept myself. I love and accept myself exactly the way I am. I still love and accept myself. Take a deep breath every time you shift tapping. Say: *"All my anger 'release'. I release the anger I have for myself. I release the anger I have for others. I release any anger I have within me. I release any anger I have about anything. I release all my anger. I release all my anger at myself. I release all my anger about life. I release all my anger about my health. I release all my anger about relationships. I release all my anger about my career. I release all my anger about my financial life. I release all my anger about anything. Even though I'm angry at myself, even though I'm angry at myself, I love and accept myself. I love and accept myself exactly the way I am."*

Now take a deep breath at last, close your eyes, think about that emotion again and give it a rating. You must be feeling better and the rating will surely drop.

It doesn't matter how long you are dealing with that emotion, it will just wash out within 5 minutes. It is worth doing at least twice a day. The important part is not to practice EFT, just generally, but to really practice EFT exactly at the time when the emotion happens. The emotion is like a baby. Do babies grow in size? Yes. Similarly, emotions also grow in size. So if you do the EFT after the baby has become this big, maybe you'll need the release technique and the EFT and the NLP and the Ho'Oponopono everything. Sometimes, when the baby is small, and you do the EFT technique, the emotion will release so fast.

Whenever there is anger (or any negative emotion) inside you, just release it at the same moment, instead of waiting for one day to release it, and then it'll be gone very easily.

If you have done it along with the reading, you must have felt a huge difference in your motions. If you do it later, you feel this at that time. Why does this happen? Your body has veins where blood is flowing through it. This blood is nothing but made of energy. Now the blood is flowing through your energy meridian points. When the blood is flowing through energy meridian points, if you've got negative emotions stored in your body, they will move out because all of these negative emotions that live in our body are made up of energy. So what happens is they go inside the blood cells of our cells and it converts into material form over there and it becomes small, small particles of blockages? The more blockages in your body, the less your blood flows properly. The more you do EFT, the more the blood flows properly again. And as a result of that, the blockages are gone.

The founder of EFT had done a beautiful research where he took a person who was a patient, kind of cancer patient, took his blood sample and put it under a microscope to check how healthy the blood cells were. If the blood cells are healthy, will they be comfortable and away from each other, or will they be like, constricted and tight against each other? They will be away from each other so that they can easily move. The same thing happens with us. We all want space.

When you constrict both your hands together, all the blood cells in your hand come together because you're constricting them together. That's exactly what's happening inside the body when there are blood cell blockages. Because of the blockages, the blood cells come together and feel difficult to move. So the founder of EFT, he took blood tests of a person who had cancer, and he saw that the blood cells came really close. But then he did a few rounds of EFT, just about three or four rounds of EFT, and then he again compared the blood test, and he found that the blood cells had just relaxed. And the more the blood cells are relaxed, the more there is healing happening in the body. Is our body capable of healing ourselves for almost anything in life? Yes, our body is blessed with the power of self healing. But sometimes when the problem is big or long, we need to stimulate it. That's exactly what EFT does.

CHAPTER 7

EMOTIONAL HEALING TECHNIQUE

"Apologize to the universe, forgive yourself, thank for the lessons, and love your existence. Ho'Oponopono is cosmic healing."

Now let's learn the next technique, which is the most important technique for healing emotions after EFT. This is the technique of NLP.

What is NLP?

Neuro-linguistic programming (NLP) is a psychological approach that uses communication, behavioral, and perceptual techniques to change someone's thoughts and behaviors. It focuses on how the mind and body influence each other through communication and our senses.

Mainly we use this technique to release physical pain like shoulder, back, neck, throat pain, etc. If you have any physical pain, give this a rating on the intensity scale. If you don't have any physical pain, check any discomfort in your body somewhere. Even the small discomforts have a lot of emotional blockages stored within that area of your body.

Now you've got that physical pain identified, give that a rating. It's a very simple technique and doesn't require music. It requires certain questions. Keep your hand on the point where you are feeling pain for a couple of seconds, if possible. Also, keep your eyes closed while doing so. And after a few seconds, you can remove your hand. You don't need to keep your hand there for too long. Now you need to give your pain a shape. It can be circular or long like a rod. And image what color is coming in your mind when you think about the pain.

Usually people say circular shape and black color. Now check if it is moving or still and if it is small or big and is it soft pain or hard??

Now I want you to change its shape to your favorite shape. If it was circular earlier, make it anything you want. If you thought of a triangle, imagine it's a beautiful triangle. Now change the color from black (previous color) to your favorite color (for example, let's take yellow). Now change its movement. If it was moving earlier, make it still. If it was still earlier, make it move. Now make its size too small. If it was large, make it small. If it was already small, make it smaller.

Imagine it as a beautiful and soft texture triangle with a beautiful yellow color. And now imagine that this triangle has converted into a beautiful balloon. Now, whatever size and shape you all have, imagine it's converted into a beautiful helium balloon which flies. And imagine that it is flying away from that part to far away in the sky. Turn your head towards the window of your room and imagine it going out of that window and becoming smaller. It keeps becoming smaller and smaller. There is some sunlight outside, and it is just melting in that sunlight and disappearing and becoming the part of sunlight. It's becoming sun energy and giving nutrients to the earth. Now open your eyes.

Now check the intensity of that pain. It must have decreased. If you do this regularly, you will find that something good is happening in your life. If you were facing financial problems before, suddenly something about your money frequency will grow because some part of the pain you were storing in your body is now released; emotionally, you'll start making some better decisions in life.

In NLP, one of the things we learn is that all emotions are lies. Because all emotions are manufactured. Emotions are not true. If emotions were the ultimate truth, then why are emotions changing every day? They're changing every day because they're not true. They're just manufactured based on our body. They're based on the way you perceive things in your mind. NLP gives us some specific techniques on how to change that perception in our mind. So pain lives in our body in a particular code. NLP gives you that code. If you change the code, the emotion changes. The code we just worked on was **"shape, color, movement, size and texture."**

NLP with Others:

Whenever you want to understand the code of any pain of anybody, just ask them to close their eyes and ask themselves the same questions: What is the current shape of your pain? What is the color? What is the movement? Is it moving or still? Is it small or big? Is it soft or hard? Most of them will always tell you hard. Now ask them to change the shape to their favorite shape. Change it to your favorite color. Change the movement, make it smaller and imagine that it has become soft like a balloon. Ask them to flee this balloon. The moment you blow the balloon, tell them to physically move their neck towards the window of their room and imagine that the pain is going out of their body, out of that window. It's going far. And the moment it's out in the sunlight, it's melted in the sunlight and becomes sunlight and merges on this earth, giving nurturing to the earth. Now quickly ask them to open their eyes. You can now ask about the new ratings again.

I guarantee you the pain will either be 70% to 80% down or zero. If the pain remains one or two, what will we do? We repeat the same process. Same can be done with emotions.

NLP for Emotions:

If you are feeling any discomfort or any emotional pain, kind of anger, hurt, sadness, anything, you can actually do NLP directly on that. First of all, ask yourself what is the negative emotion you are suffering from (it can be any emotion, but I am assuming it is 'Fear'). We always feel every emotion in a certain part of our body. So check where you are feeling the emotion? Is it in your heart? Is it in your stomach? Is it in your head? Is it in your legs? Let's assume the stomach. Now, what is the level of the emotion? On the scale of one to ten.

Now we have all the details of that emotion, so let's start healing this.

Close your eyes and think about the cause of that emotion. If it was fear, think of something that scares you. Keep your eyes and check where in your body does that pain reside? In our example above, it's the stomach. Now think about the shape and color of that pain. For example, it can be circle and red. Imagine its movement and size and texture.

Now change the shape and color to your choice. Let's change it to oval and sky blue. Now change its movement. If it was still earlier, think it's moving now and if it was moving earlier, make it still. Now make it small and imagine it's becoming smaller and smaller, like a dot. Make it beautiful and soft. Now convert it into a balloon. Imagine a beautiful sky blue (color of your choice) oval shaped (shape of your choice) balloon flying away from that body part towards the sun through your room window. Move your head towards the window of your room and imagine it's going out of your body and your stomach towards the window. It's gone out of the window. Now it's going far. It's becoming a small dot. And it's merging in the sunlight and disappearing and becoming sunlight and going on the earth and nurturing the earth. Now quickly open your eyes and divert your mind on something else. And now check your fear quickly in your stomach. Ask yourself all questions again and give this a rating. You will find that the rating is now low. Now you can repeat the process again and decrease the rating to zero.

CHAPTER 8

RELEASE TECHNIQUE

"In the simplicity of 'I'm sorry, please forgive me, thank you, I love you,' Ho'Oponopono unfolds its profound healing magic." – Morrnah Nalamaku Simeona

This chapter is about the release technique. Release technique is a specific technique of a series of questions. The more you ask these questions in the same sequence, you will let something released from your body. For example, let me tell you about the story of one of my clients. She had some marks on her body. Some on hands and some on feet and neck as well. Slowly, the marks started spreading all over the body.

And obviously, if there are so many marks on your body, you start getting a little bit scared. So she consulted a doctor and took a lot of medicine. But medicine was not helping. Then I suggested that she do the release technique. And it worked. All of her marks disappeared from her body.

In the release technique, you take a seat at one place. And as you start the release technique, the first question, the first statement that you say is: "Even though I am feeling this feeling physically or emotionally, consciously or unconsciously, wherever in my body, I am willing to release it." The first part is taking responsibility for wherever this feeling is coming from. It doesn't matter whether it's coming from physical symptoms or from emotional symptoms. The first question you're asking yourself is: "am I willing to release it?" That's question number one. We also do EFT along with saying the statements; you need to keep tapping on the side of your palm while saying the statement. You can do this for whatever you are feeling. Even though you may be feeling sadness, even though you may be feeling a headache, even though you may be feeling tense, even though you may be feeling worried, different people have different emotions in different situations. But whatever you are feeling at that point in time, you're asking yourself: "am I willing to release this?" Once you are ready to release this, you ask yourself: am I ready? You answer yourself: Yes, I am ready!! The moment you say 'yes', you are supposed to take a deep breath and exhale. When you exhale, you need to imagine that the pain in that part of your body or the emotion is just releasing either through your mouth or from that part of your body where there's some kind of pain.

For example, if you've got a backache, you're going to say: "even though I have this backache right now, physically or emotionally, whatever is causing this backache, consciously or unconsciously, am I willing to release it?" You say 'YES' with a deep breath and exhale. And you imagine that the backache is disappearing from your body.

The second question is the same statement with should, "should I release it?" So the first part is, "am I willing to release it?" Second question is: should I release it? Third question is "when will I release it?" In the third question, the answer is not 'yes or no'; the answer to the third question is 'NOW'. This works best when it is physical pain.

Let's understand this further with an example. Think about the physical pain you have in your body. It can be any kind of physical pain like headache, backache, shoulder pain or any kind of symptom. I am assuming someone has a leg injury. And the intensity of pain is 9, and the pain has been there for the last 24 hours. So first of all, you need to identify the pain, rate its intensity, and remember for how long you are experiencing this pain.

Generally, when we do the release technique, it's good to touch your hand over there. So in our case, the person needs to touch his/her leg. We don't have to close our eyes on this technique.

So touch that part of your body and say: *"Whatever is causing this pain in my life, whatever is causing this pain in my leg, physically or emotionally, consciously or unconsciously. Am I willing to release this pain? Say: Yes!"* You need to say 'yes' loudly and then take a deep breath. After this, imagine the pain is disappearing from your leg [body] as you exhale. Imaging this is going out of your leg [body part] like fumes.

Keep that hand on that part of your body and say: *"Whatever is causing this pain, physically or emotionally, consciously or unconsciously, should I release it? Say: Yes."* Take a deep breath. And once again, imagine that the pain is going out of that part of your leg like fumes in the air.

Touch that part of your body again and say: *"Whatever is causing this pain, whatever is little bit left, physically or emotionally, consciously or unconsciously. When will I release this? Say 'Now'."* take a deep breath and imagine the pain going out.

Now check the level of your pain, move that part of your body, and check the intensity of pain you are feeling now. The intensity must have dropped. The technique will not take over 3 to 4 minutes and you find that you are feeling way much better than you were feeling three minutes ago.

Example 2:

Let's do this for the cold and cough. For this, we need to put our hand either on our throat or on our nose. Wherever we're feeling the maximum discomfort. We will rate its intensity and will remember its duration.

While keeping the hand on the throat or nose, say: "Whatever is causing this pain, physically or emotionally, consciously or unconsciously, whatever is the reason, am I willing to release it?" say: Yes! Take a deep breath and imagine it going out from that part like fumes.

Keep the hand on that body part and say: "Whatever is causing this pain, physically or emotionally, consciously or unconsciously, whatever is the reason, should I release it?" say: Yes! You can take a sip of water. Now the last time say: *"Whatever is causing this pain, whatever is little bit left, physically or emotionally, consciously or unconsciously. When will I release this? Say 'Now'."* take a deep breath and imagine the pain going out.

After this, think about the pain and give it a rating now. The rating must have dropped. You can do the same exercise for any kind of pain, at any intensity. The same exercise can be done for emotions as well.

Exercise on behalf of others:

The exercise can be done on behalf of others. We can do the exercise to heal someone else. For this, we only need to make slight changes in the statement. We need to mention the person's name when we will recite the statements. For example, we are doing for a lady who is suffering from a cough and cold.

Put your hands on your throat and say: *"on behalf of [name] whatever is causing this pain in our neck physically or emotionally, consciously or unconsciously, am I willing to release it? Answer: yes."* now say the second statement: *"Whatever is causing the pain, physically or emotionally, unconsciously or consciously on behalf of [name], should I release this pain? Say; yes."* Now take a deep breath and imagine something is going out of her throat. Something is going out of your throat as well. One last time say: *"Whatever is stuck in our throat, whatever little bit is left, physically or emotionally, consciously or unconsciously, on behalf of [name] when will I release it? Say: Now."* And take a deep breath and imagine some white fumes going out of your throat.

The technique works the same way even if someone else is doing this for us because, at the energy level, we are all connected. We all can talk with each other and can help each other at the energy level. When we release a negative emotion within us, it gets released within that person as well. That is why I always say, **"the more you heal yourself, the more you heal others."**

If you go to a doctor and say you healed yourself or someone else within five minutes without the medicine, it will be very difficult for doctors to believe that, but they are not wrong because they come from the world of logic and we are experiencing the world of art and magic.

Now I want you to try it on somebody in your family and friends and let's see what happens. Because, as a healer, your best confidence comes not only when you heal yourself, but also when you heal other people.

CHAPTER 9

REMOTE HEALING TECHNIQUE

*"Release the past, embrace the present.
Ho'Oponopono is the spiritual art
of living in the now with love and
gratitude."*

Before we move further, I want you to start doing advanced conversational Ho'Oponopono for your mom and dad separately.

So first do it for your mom. You would start with the statement: *"I take 100% responsibility for everything that I am feeling and everything that my mom is feeling. Because at the energy level, we are all one."* And then say those statements: I'm sorry. And then give three-four reasons for why you're saying sorry to mom. Then say- Please forgive me. And give three-four statements, after this say- Thank you and I love you and give three statements for the same. You can keep going on a little more if you need to end with I'm sorry, please forgive me, thank you, I love you. And make sure that you take a deep breath at the end of it. Then do the same thing for your father.

After that, we'll use the remote healing technique directly for our parents. One feeling I always get when I do advanced conversation Ho'Oponopono for my mom and dad is I feel grounded and very relaxed. I feel like I'm home and I feel like there's no desperation. Everything looks complete. It's difficult to describe. There's a sense of balance that you feel and you know you're taken care of because you're doing Ho'oponopono with them. I want you to promise me you will do this twice a day, once in the morning, once in the night.

Remote Healing Technique:

Now let's learn about a remote healing technique. The remote healing technique is all about taking a person's photograph, keeping it in front of you in the east direction of your house. So generally either you should use a compass or you could use a mobile application for determining the direction. Once you have the compass, look at where the east direction of your room is. It's good to keep that photograph standing or you can place it against the East wall. When we do direct energetic healing with anybody, the results are actually ten times faster than just having a conversation with anybody.

The first step is to take a photograph and go in the east direction. Best is to keep it on the wall or on a table. Make sure the photograph is stable and don't hold it. Then we look at the photograph and use the technique which we are going to learn.

Let's take a hypothetical person having some back pain. And the intensity of this pain is 8 or 9, which means the level of pain is very high. We will start by doing advanced Ho'Oponopono for this person. You can get the music rolling. Keep your hands on your heart and say: *"I take 100% responsibility on behalf of [Name of the person]. Because I am [his/her name]. Because at the energy level, we are one. I am sorry on behalf of [Name] for doing whatever I have done to cause this pain in my body. Please forgive me, I'm really sorry for doing whatever I have done to cause this pain in [Name]'s body. I'm really sorry for holding on to some emotions which are creating pain. It is just my emotions because many times during the same pain, I'm fine. Please forgive me. Please forgive me for not taking responsibility. Please forgive me for constantly worrying about my backache. Please forgive me for not taking responsibility. Thank you, my dear body, for taking care of me even though I have trouble listening to you now. Whatever is creating the pain in our body, physically or emotionally, I am willing to release it on behalf of [Name]."*

Now take a deep breath and release the pain the same as we did in EFT. Imagine that energy is going out of your back and the person's back. This time, touch your back, and say: *"Whatever is causing this pain in my back as [Name], physically or emotionally, consciously or unconsciously, I will release it."* Take a deep breath and release it. Imagine that energy has just gone out of your back.

Everyone has to experience pain; it's the nature of our body and a proof that we are living beings. But it is a limiting belief that you have to be disturbed during that time. You may have realized there are certain times when you're completely fine in spite of the pain. Sometimes you are in pain, but emotionally, you're completely fine. That's why the pain is actually a limiting belief. The pain is not in your body, it's in your emotional pattern. We have learned before that all emotions are lies; it's all an emotional pattern. And if you learn to change your patterns, it doesn't matter what body patterns you're going through, you can change your feelings.

I remember one of my friends who was going through sciatica; he had sciatica for approximately nine months. And in spite of the pain in his back, he used to do workshops. And his backache in those days was so bad that if he walked for even 10ft, he had to lie down after that for five minutes; it was that bad. And in spite of that, when he did the workshops, guess what his physical strength was? To stand fully upright. He used to stand and deliver the workshop. That means **"all emotions are lies."** It's possible for you to take control of your emotions, irrelevant of what you're going through your body.

CHAPTER 10

SOLVING UNIVERSAL PROBLEM USING HO'OPONOPONO WISDOM

*"In the silence of forgiveness, we find
the true music of the heart."
- Dr. Ihaleakalá Hew Len*

In this chapter, we're going to learn once again about Ho'Oponopono. In previous chapters, we've already learned about Ho'Oponopono. Briefly, what is the law of attraction? Law of attraction works on the science of words. It believes that words have energy and frequency. Ho'Oponopono is made of four statements:

1. I'm sorry,

2. Please forgive me.

3. Thank you.

4. I love you.

The first basis of Ho'Oponopono is having positive vibrations. Like: "I'm sorry, please forgive me, thank you and I love you. You can use these positive vibrations to heal anything in your life. Any negative energy can be cleaned out from your life for somebody else, for yourself. Using Ho'Oponopono with these four statements, the second basis on which the law of attraction works or Ho'Oponopono works is on the basis that it takes 100% responsibility. We take 100% responsibility for everything in our life. Suppose if my daughter is feeling bad about something, I don't go and heal her in Ho'Oponopono. I just simply do Ho'Oponopono for myself and I take 100% responsibility for that. Ho'Oponopono always starts with the simple way *"I take 100% responsibility for what I'm feeling right now. I'm sorry. Please forgive me. Thank you. I love you."* Same thing can be done when you're doing it for others.

Some of the most asked questions:

Question: The most common question asked to me is how do you do it?

When you are doing Ho'Oponopono for somebody else. Actually, you are not doing Ho'Oponopono for somebody else. You are doing this for yourself.

- Once my student asked me a question, she wanted to do Ho'Oponopono for her sister. And she was upset about something between sister and her. She can do Ho'Oponopono for her sister by saying: I'm sorry, [sister's name], please forgive me. I love you. Thank you. You can do this for any person you are having troubles with.

- Once I met a gentleman who asked me a question. He and his mother had some challenges. He was saying, what should I do? Why does she behave like this? I told him to do Ho'Oponopono. I told him to take full responsibility for what happened between you and your mom. Once you start taking complete responsibility for it, then you chant "I'm sorry mom. Please forgive me. I love you. Thank you." and you will find that the problem is resolved. You have to exit the blame mode and start taking the responsibility. Responsibility is very important. If you take the responsibility, then these affirmations actually work. If you don't take the responsibility and then chant for the sake of it then it will not work.

Question: Next question is how to do Ho'Oponopono for negative thinking?

If you are thinking negatively, then just take full responsibility. You can say: "I'm thinking negatively. I'm sorry about that. So I'm sorry. Please forgive me. I love you. Thank you." It's a very simple technique.

So whenever a negative thought (worry, fear, anxiety etc.) comes into my mind, I just simply catch myself, stop myself and chant I'm sorry, please forgive me, I love you. For that particular emotion or thought. I do this till the time my monkey mind doesn't wander somewhere else and finish up.

This works best when you do it for 108 times. It is a magic number. This can also be done eleven times.

Question: How to do this to find a new job?

First, identify if you already know the employer. If not, you just say that "I'm sorry. The new employer. Please forgive me. I love you. You can also do it for yourself- "I'm sorry, Please forgive me, I love you, thank you." Because you are taking the ownership of not having a job or losing a job or being in the situation where you don't have a job.

You can also do it for the anxiety that you are getting in the job.

Whenever you are doing Ho'Oponopono, don't use logic too much, just chant the affirmations and it works. Do you use logic when you are sweeping your house? When you're cleaning your house? You just take the broom in the morning and you just start cleaning. As simple as that. Do you think you should start from the left side of your house or the right side of your house? Should you broom it three or four times or should you broom it or not?

Question: How to do this for a broken relationship in friendship?

First, take the ownership of that broken relationship. That means that the relationship is broken. And you take full responsibility for what went wrong between you and your friend.

Question: How to do Ho'Oponopono for broken relationship between siblings?

Take responsibility for what happened between you and your sibling. Second, stop judging your sibling. When you take full responsibility for what has happened between you and your sibling, you will stop judging him/her and stop blaming him/her. Once you do that, then you chant for him/her. Whatever is their name, I'm assuming Monika is her name. "I will say I'm sorry, Monika. Please forgive me. I love you. Thank you." And you need to do that for five days. And in these five days, don't blame your sibling for anything. Don't judge him/her. You will see a dramatic difference between your relationships with them.

Question: How to do this to get pregnant?

For pregnancy, there are a few things. Take a water bottle, put a sticker written: "Hey, I'm pregnant. I'm going to deliver a baby...." this type of lines. And put a vision board with the pregnancy photo and put whatever affirmations you want on it. And whenever you get worried during the day about the pregnancy, don't get worried. Say, I'm going to have a baby. Do the Ho'Oponopono. You can say: "I'm sorry, my child. Please forgive me. I love you. Thank you." And also do affirmations as if you've already got the child.

When you create a perfect frequency, the attraction happens faster. Without affirmations, it doesn't mean that only Ho'Oponopono will attract something. Ho'Oponopono is not a tuner to tune your frequency. It is to clean the frequency. So that when you do the tuning, it works.

If you're in a house where you've got a phone call and the range is not coming. Sometimes you go to the balcony and the range comes in. Because you've opened up all blockages when you go to the balcony. And now the frequency is reaching directly to you on the phone. And the phone is working. That is what we are doing with Ho'Oponopono. We're removing all the blockages. So your frequency works, your affirmations work. Try to do affirmations, do water bottle, vision boards, everything.

Question: How to heal patients with Ho'Oponopono?

If someone is suffering from severe diseases like diabetes and no medication is working, we can heal them with Ho'Oponopono. You can do: "I'm sorry [name of patient]. Please forgive me. I love you. Thank you." While doing that, visualize that he/she is healthy and fit.

Question: How to apply this technique to get PR for Canada?

You can do water bottle, do vision board that you are already in Canada. Along with that, say: "I'm sorry, Canada. Please forgive me. I love you. Thank you."

Just catch the emotion and replace it with Ho'Oponopono. This is a standard rule for any worry, any fear, anxiety you are having during the day. Catch it and say "I'm sorry. Please forgive me. I love you. Thank you."

Question: How to do Ho'Oponopono for hearing loss and weak eyesight?

You can say: "I'm sorry, please forgive me. I love you. Thank you for making me absolutely healthy and fit. And also for any negative emotion about health."

Let me tell you about my friend. He made more than $10,000 selling a property. He purchased a property in the US. He purchased it for $10,000 and within a month he put it on sale. He created a vision board and started visualizing that it is sold for $20,000. And he started chanting: "I'm sorry, (property name). Please forgive me. I love you. Thank you." That's all he did. Within a month, he sold his house for $20,000 and made a huge profit.

Question: What image should be there in our mind when we chant Ho'Oponopono?

You should visualize your goals; you should imagine yourself completing the goal.

There is a friend of mine once she dropped one bottle full of water on her Mac air. It was a brand new Mac air, only six months old; obviously it was a painful experience for her. So she and I both decided to do

Ho'Oponopono. I sincerely did 108 Ho'Oponopono for that Mac air. And she also did. We both manifested that the Mac air is working. Believe it or not, the Mac air started working. It's unbelievable, it's a miracle.

Another friend of mine lost her car keys, and she was not able to get them. She just generally called me and she told me, we both did the Ho'Oponopono and she instantly found the keys in her bag. So I always do this for my appliances, for my robots, for my laptops, gadgets for everything. This works because this is energy. We are also energy. You can communicate with it and it works.

Let's see how to use Ho'Oponopono for few more Day-to-Day Problems

Everything in the universe is made of frequency. And our words that we use are also made of frequency. For example, when you sing a song, the vibrations of that song become part of your emotions, become part of your mood. Once that becomes part of your mood, whatever your frequency you're vibrating at, you start attracting that in your life. When you sing energetic songs, you feel energetic, but if you start singing sad songs; you start attracting negative things in your life. Ho'Oponopono works on the same science of sound and vibrations and energy.

Four statements that Dr. Hew Len has discovered are: I am sorry, please forgive me, thank you, I love you. These are very humble statements. So the frequency is beautiful. The frequency is very humble. When you say I'm sorry, please forgive me. Your frequency becomes very humble, very down to earth. When you say thank you, I love you; you are adding gratitude to your nature. Frequency of "I love you" is love frequency. When you start repeating these four statements again and again, it creates a beautiful vibration inside you, a wonderful frequency inside you, which then clears out any negative energy inside you. And as a result of that, you start attracting positive frequency. Your affirmations start working. This is Ho'Oponopono.

In this section, we are going to understand how you can use Ho'Oponopono for multiple things with the help of questions asked by my clients.

Question: How to do Ho'Oponopono to achieve our dream college?

Answer: A lot of people think that they are supposed to use Ho'Oponopono to attract something. Which is not correct. The way you're supposed to do it is first you do an affirmation that says thank you, universe. I have already attracted my dream college. I'm already studying in my dream college. It's been more than one month I'm studying here and I'm loving the campus. I'm having a great relationship with my new friends. Immediately after that, say Ho'Oponopono. So that whatever doubt that comes in you about attracting that college clears up because of Ho'Oponopono. Say: I'm sorry, please forgive me, thank you. I love you immediately after saying that affirmation. If you say it even before the affirmation becomes more powerful. Why does it become more powerful? Because before you're saying the affirmation, you're going through some doubt. When you say I'm sorry, please forgive me. Thank you, I love you. You're clearing out the doubts. Then you're saying the affirmation. Both sides affirmation in between becomes perfect frequency as a result of which you start attracting your goals.

Question: How to use it for a relation?

Answer: Let's say you want to use Ho'Oponopono for your relationship with your father. And you and your father are not getting along well. All you have to do is- think about your father and say, dad, I'm sorry. Please forgive me. Thank you. I love you. The thumb rule here is when you're doing Ho'Oponopono for that person, do it 108 times. If you really are doing it for relationships, whenever you want Ho'Oponopono frequency to go really powerful, do it 108 times. Think about that person and 108 times repeat these whole four statements. I'm sorry. Please forgive me. Thank you. I love you. If you do it twice a day, any negative energy between you and that person then disappears. Then you can even do affirmations after this that my father and I are getting along really well. We have a wonderful relationship. And my father and I are sitting together, having dinner together. He's laughing, I'm laughing. We both are having a wonderful relationship. Once again, say I'm sorry, dad. Please forgive me. Thank you. I love you.

Question: How to do this for negative things or situations?

Answer: Hypothetically, if you are under a home loan, you can do Ho'Oponopono. You can say: my home loan I'm sorry for feeling bad for you. Please forgive me. Thank you dear home loan, for having been in my life. I love you dear home loan, I'm sorry dear loan. Please forgive me dear loan for feeling bad about you. Thank you, dear loan for giving me the benefits of the money that you have given me. I love you dear loan for everything that you have given me in my life. Because of this, the purpose of that loan gets cleared. Now you get the positive energy to create money to be able to clear off that loan. And as a result of that, the loan goes away in your life.

Question: How to deal with medical problems with it?

Answer: One of my clients' cousins was two and a half years old and could not speak. Doctors say it's a mild case of autism. To heal this type of situation, what you can do is take a photograph of your cousin. Especially works very well for children. Take a photograph and do it early in the morning. When you wake up, do Ho'Oponopono 108 times. Also, do it at night when he's going to sleep completely. About 1 hour after that. Why? Because after 1 hour he goes deep into sleep. When he's deep in sleep, his conscious mind is no more interfering with you. His subconscious mind has opened up at the energy level. Now when you look at his photograph and you say Ho'Oponopono 108 times, it becomes even more powerful. And you'll see that whatever negative energy is there between you and him, not only that will clear up, he will start getting positive vibrations. As a result of that, you will see him having a much healthier mindset. Dr. Hew Len had done this in his mental hospital, with mental patients who were criminally psychotic people. He used Ho'Oponopono on them every single day for many months, for about six months. And as a result of that, he was able to cure all of them. And literally, that mental hospital had closed down. That is why Ho'Oponopono became so famous. So if Dr. Hew Len can do that, why can't we?

I'm not saying this is my medical opinion. I'm not a doctor, so I can't say that. But I'm telling you, using Ho'Oponopono's story, Dr. Hew Len's story, that if he can do it, what harm is it to at least try? The only thing is consistency is required. Don't do it for one day and expect amazing results the next day. And then stop having hopes. Use it every single day for months and months and months. You'll start seeing positive benefits because, at the energy level, you're transferring a lot of positive energy to the patient. So do it in the morning, do it in the night after he sleeps, if you can even touch him and do it at night. If you stay with him, if he stays with you, if you can touch him and do it when he's sleeping at night, you will get even better results.

Question: How to attract a job in a desired company using hope?

Answer: I always say that don't try to attract a job in a particular company that blocks your frequency. Why does it block your frequency? Maybe the universe wants to give you a better job. But you're behind the universe saying I want a job only from this company. There are chances of contradiction between you and the universe. So, never make affirmation for a particular type of company. Always say thank you, universe. I am now working in my dream company. I'm so happy working here. It's been more than one month, and my first salary is already deposited into my account. And the best part is, I have an amazing relationship with my boss, my colleagues, and I'm having a lot of work satisfaction here. This is the affirmation that you should have before saying this affirmation. Say Ho'Oponopono after saying this affirmation. Any doubt that you may have while saying the affirmation will clear up because you're saying Ho'Oponopono immediately after saying the Ho'Oponopono. After the affirmation, if you say Ho'Oponopono again, which is, I'm sorry, please forgive me. Thank you. I love you. Any negative block which might be stopping that job from being attracted to you will also get cleared up. You can also say this: thank you, universe. I've got my dream job now in an amazing bank. I'm so happy working here. I have an amazing relationship with my boss and my work satisfaction is so much. I'm loving every day that I work in this bank. Thank you, universe. I am so happy working in this bank. I'm sorry. Please forgive me. Thank you. I love you. Now you repeat, I'm sorry. Please forgive me. Thank you. I love you. About eleven times after you say the affirmation, it helps clear any negative energy that you have or doubt that you have about that affirmation.

Question: How to do it for height?

Answer: I would say instead of doing it for height, do it for your confidence that I'm sorry for the way I feel about myself. Please forgive me. Thank you for my personal confidence. I love my confidence. I love myself the way I am now. If you are 15 years old, then obviously height can work for you. Then you can simply say: I'm sorry for feeling bad about my height. Please forgive me for having tension for my height. Thank you so much, universe. I am now 6ft tall. I love myself the way I am. You can do this when you're 15, 16, or 17 years old. But once you cross 18, you're going against the laws of the universe. After this age, it doesn't work. If you're beyond 18, instead of doing it for height, start doing it for your confidence. Start doing it for your self esteem. You want to be tall because you want to be impressive in front of people, but you can only be impressive in front of other people when you're impressed by yourself. If you are 6ft tall and you're not impressed with yourself, even height will not solve that problem. So always do affirmation directly for the end result of your self confidence and then say I'm sorry for feeling bad about my height. I'm sorry for feeling bad about my personality. Please forgive me. Thank you for my amazing personality, for my confident personality. I love myself the way I am.

Question: How to do it for having a child?

Answer: you can start doing Ho'Oponopono with thinking of your wife and your upcoming child and say thank you, my dear child. I'm sorry, my dear child, for feeling low and confident about having you in my life. Please forgive me. Thank you, my dear child, for being in my life. I love you, my dear child, for coming into my life and into my family. You must do Ho'Oponopono twice a day, 108 times for your child and for your wife. Other than that you can also use the water bottle technique which says my child is happy, healthy and dancing in my family. Write this affirmation on the water bottle. Keep this water bottle filled next to you all night. When you wake up in the morning, drink water from this. Your wife should also drink water from this and finish this water in 2 to 3 hours. Do this every night. There are so many people I have already got results from who have said that by using the water bottle technique, they've got a child in their family. It's possible, but your frequency, your feeling needs to be comfortable and peaceful. And for that, you should use Ho'Oponopono twice a day for your baby.

Question: How to do this if the relationship is at a very bad stage?

Answer: Take his/her photograph, look at his photo twice a day and do Ho'Oponopono 108 times. The affirmation that you should do is 'thank you, universe. We are back together. We are very happy together. Thank you, universe, for a wonderful relationship between me and him/her.' This part will definitely work which is doing Ho'Oponopono for him/her. Any negative frequency between you and him will disappear. But because of the way you have energy, you have frequency. He/she also has energy and frequency and matching of these two energies is a very important thing. So the best way to do it is to do better affirmations for your end result, which is: thank you, universe. I'm happily married now. I'm very happy with my wonderful life partner who is an amazing life partner. I love my life partner. My life partner loves me. This is the end result of affirmation. If you do this end result affirmation, maybe he/she will get attracted to you. Maybe someone better will get attracted to you. But at least the stress in your life about that person will move away. And as a result of that, attraction happens. Maybe through him/her, maybe through another person. You have to trust the universe and surrender to the universe for that.

Question: How to do Ho'Oponopono for a son/daughter/student who is about to appear for the CA intermediate exam?

Answer: you can start with the affirmations like: I'm sorry for feeling tense about my son and his exams. Please forgive me. Thank you, universe. My son has already passed a CA exam. I love my son for passing his CA exams. So you combine your affirmation and Ho'Oponopono here once again, Do this about 108 times, morning and evening and then see the magic. Most importantly, if your son can also do the same affirmation with mixed Ho'Oponopono, you will get brilliant results.

Question: How to attract a life partner?

Answer: You can say: I'm sorry for feeling stressed without a partner. Please forgive me for feeling stressed without a partner in my life. Thank you, universe, for giving me this life. I love myself the way I am. I have an amazing life partner. I have been happily married for over three months now. We have a wonderful relationship. I'm getting along with my in-laws. My in-laws are thrilled with me. Thank you, universe, for a very, very happy married life. I'm sorry, universe, for doubting you earlier. Thank you; please forgive me the universe for feeling stressed about this marriage. Thank you so much universe. I am happily married now. I love being happily married to my wonderful life partner. So you can see that we said Ho'Oponopono just before and after the affirmations. Say it again and again twice a day, 108 times, and see the magic happening.

CONCLUSION

Congratulations on reaching the culmination of this book. Your commitment to reading through these pages signifies your dedication to personal growth and a thirst for knowledge. Completing a book is a remarkable achievement, and you should take a moment to acknowledge your accomplishment.

Throughout this journey, the aim has been to guide you toward shaping a destiny defined by success and fulfillment. Your investment in this book reflects a deep commitment to self-improvement, and for that, you should feel proud.

As you conclude this book, I trust that it has left you with valuable insights and a sense of empowerment. The road to a prosperous destiny is not always linear or without its challenges, but your newfound knowledge in smart questioning equips you to navigate these paths with confidence. I genuinely hope that your voyage through these chapters has been both enlightening and engaging. The pursuit of a splendid life brimming with happiness and fulfillment is a commendable one, and your proactive steps toward this aspiration are evident through your persistence in reading this book.

In the pursuit of success and a life well-lived, remember that knowledge is your most potent tool. With this, you hold the key to unlocking the limitless potential within you. As you close this final page and embark on the journey that follows, I extend my heartfelt best wishes for a future filled with accomplishments and contentment.

Cheers,
Sooraj Achar

MAY I ASK YOU FOR A SMALL FAVOR?

I want to express my sincere gratitude for choosing to invest your time in reading this book. Your decision to explore this work among countless others means a lot to me.

I hope that within these pages, you've discovered actionable insights that can enhance your daily life. Your journey doesn't have to end here, though.

May I kindly request an additional 30 seconds of your valuable time?

Sharing your thoughts about the book through a review would be immensely appreciated. Your review serves as a beacon, guiding other readers to take a chance on my books. It's a small gesture that carries significant weight in the world of authors.

To submit your review effortlessly, please **Scan** the **QR Code** below. It will take you directly to the book's review page:

"The Alchemy of Healing" or "Global Link"

Alternatively, you can also find the "**Reviews Section**" of this book's page on Amazon.

Your review will require just a minute of your time but will make a monumental difference in helping me connect with a broader audience and I eagerly look forward to reading your review.

Once again, thank you for your unwavering support of my work.

PREVIEW OF MY BEST SELLING BOOKS

Series-1: Master Your Life with NUMEROLOGY

★ **Why do 80% of People Fail to Recognize their True Potential ??**

These self-help books will help you **Recognize, Transform, and Navigate** your life toward a **Happier Destiny**.

I always say that your **Date of Birth** is so precious. God has placed many diamonds on your date of birth that you are not aware of. It doesn't matter if your date of birth is good or bad. The idea is how you can take the best out of your date of birth. **Master Your DESTINY With Numerology** is a perfect, **complete beginner's guide** for those who are new to numerology.

★ What Role Does Numerology Play in Your Life?

- You have been surrounded by numbers since the day you were Born. Now use them to unlock your Destiny.

- Wherever you go in your life, the numbers always move on with you.

- When you are born, on the very first day of your life, you get your date of birth, which is made up of numbers.

- When you get admitted to school, you get your roll number.

- When you get your results, you get a percentage of numbers.

- When you get a job, you get a salary and EMP-ID number.

- When you buy any vehicle, it has a number plate.

- When you travel, you get a ticket and seat number

- When you check into a hotel, you get a room number.

- When you want to call a person, you have to dial numbers.

- When you get married, there is also a date attached to it.

- If there is Life, there are Numbers. You cannot get rid of Numbers.

★ Your **Name Spelling** also plays an important role according to your date of birth. Believe me or not, **30% to 40%** of your success or failure depends on your name spelling. If you keep your name spelling correct, you can achieve 30% to 40% more success in your life.

♥ **Master Your DESTINY With Numerology will help you...**

✓ Recognize Your Strengths and Weaknesses.

✓ Find Your Lucky Numbers and Colors.

✓ Correct Your Name Spelling without changing your documents.

✓ Choose the Right Profession.

✓ Find a Compatible Life-Partner.

✓ With Simple Remedies for All Your Problems.

✓ Check Your Foreign or Abroad Opportunities.

✓ Predict your Future Years, Months, and Days of importance, which helps you make Better Decisions.

✓ Understand the Behavioral Patterns of People Around You.

✓ Transform and Navigate your life for a Better Future.

★ If you are ready to make a commitment to yourself that you want to learn everything that is presented to you, then it is our commitment to you that this will surely help you a lot. There is no reason why this book will not change your destiny or transform your future. But, there is an important thing you must keep in mind, i.e., **"You will bring this change through TRANSFORMATION, not through MIRACLES".**

★ If you learn **Numerology**, then

(a) "You will be **awakened**", which makes it likely to "**transform**" your life.

(b) Ultimately, "You will be able to **navigate** your life".

★ Life is all about "**Awakening**,", "**Transformation**," and eventually, "Knowing How To **Navigate** It?"

★ Order **Master Your DESTINY With Numerology** now to make the most of your **Health, Relationships, Career, and Money** by unlocking the **Power of Numbers.**

Check Out My Best Selling Books Here:

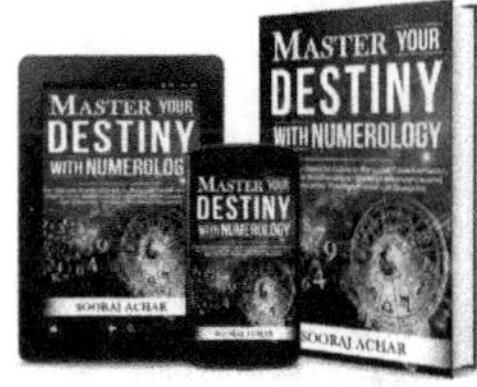

1. Master Your DESTINY With Numerology

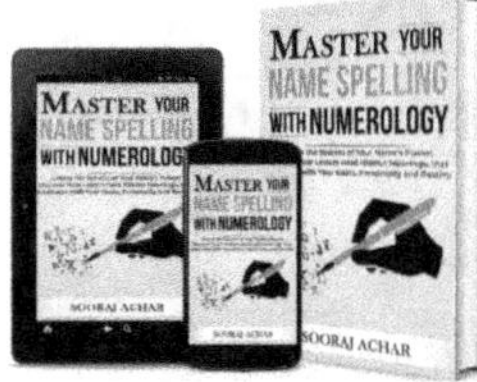

2. Master Your NAME-SPELLING With Numerology

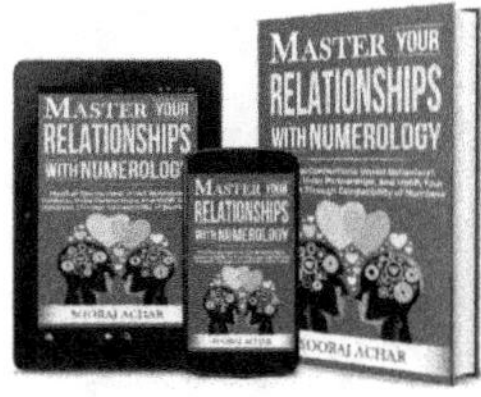

3. Master Your RELATIONSHIPS With Numerology

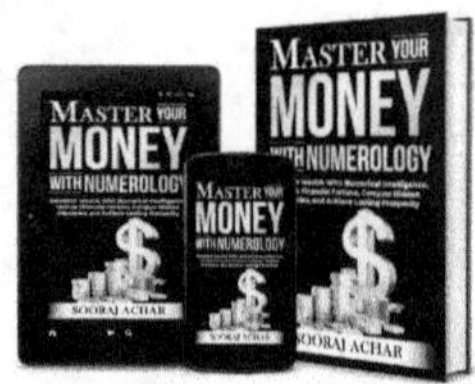

4. Master Your MONEY With Numerology

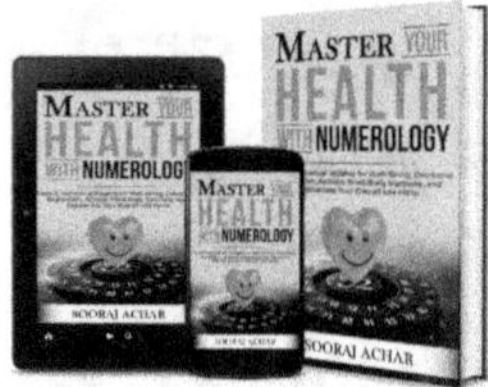

5. Master Your HEALTH With Numerology

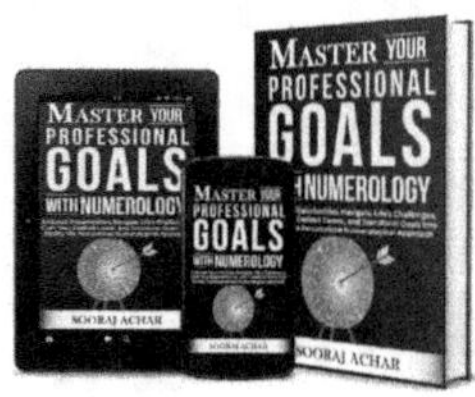

6. Master Your PROFESSIONAL GOALS With Numerology

Series-2: Master Your Life with VASTU

★ How Can These Books Work Miracles in Your Life?

This Self-Help Book is A Perfect Blueprint Describing Ancient Principles for Modern Living. A Step-by-step Practical Guide for Beginners to Creating a Positive Living Space and for Optimal Well-Being.

Learn:

★ How to Implement Feng-Shui/Vastu in your Day-to-Day Life !!

★ What Role Do Feng-Shui and Vastu Play in Your Life?

★ Relationship between Vastu and Feng-Shui?

Vastu is used to Diagnose, and Feng Shui is the Remedy. Vastu is used to identify the disease, and Feng Shui is the medicine. Vastu and Feng Shui are complementary to each other.

Vastu Shastra is an Ancient Indian Science of architecture and construction, which is based on the principles of harmony and balance between humans and their environment. The main focus of Vastu is to create a harmonious balance between the 5-Elements of nature, i.e., Earth, Water, Air, Fire, & Space. It emphasizes directions and orientation and uses various elements like colors, shapes, and materials to create a balance and positive energy in the living spaces.

Feng Shui, on the other hand, is a Chinese Philosophical System of harmonizing everyone with the surrounding environment. It is based on the principles of Qi (Chi), the life force that flows through all living things, and Yin and Yang, the balance of opposite forces. Feng Shui focuses on the placement of objects, furniture, and structures in living spaces to optimize the flow of energy, or "Qi." It also considers the orientation of the building, the placement of doors and windows, and the use of colors, shapes, & materials to create balance & harmony.

In summary, both Vastu and Feng Shui aim to create balance and harmony in living spaces, but Vastu is more focused on directions and orientation, while Feng Shui emphasizes the flow of energy & balance of opposing forces.

★ The Benefits of Reading This Book Include:

✓ **Health and Well-Being:** Vastu principles aim to create a harmonious and balanced environment that can promote physical, mental, and emotional well-being.

✓ **Financial Prosperity:** Vastu principles are believed to help attract positive energy and good fortune, leading to financial prosperity.

✓ **Improved Relationships:** Vastu principles can help create an atmosphere of peace and harmony, which can lead to improved relationships with family, friends, & colleagues.

✓ **Increased Productivity:** A Vastu-compliant environment is said to be conducive to productivity and efficiency, leading to greater success in personal & professional life.

✓ **Spiritual Growth:** Vastu principles are based on ancient Vedic knowledge and aim to promote spiritual growth & enlightenment.

✓ **Enhanced Creativity:** Vastu principles are believed to enhance creativity and inspiration, which can be beneficial for artists, writers, & other creative professionals.

✓ **Better Sleep Quality:** Vastu principles can help create a peaceful and relaxing environment, which can improve the quality of sleep and help reduce stress & anxiety.

✓ **Improved Mental Clarity:** A Vastu-compliant environment is said to help clear the mind and improve mental clarity, which can be beneficial for decision-making & problem-solving.

✓ **Enhanced Career Prospects:** Vastu principles can help align one's career goals with their personal strengths and abilities, leading to greater career success & satisfaction.

★ Overall, the benefits of Vastu can contribute to a more Balanced, Harmonious, & Fulfilling Life.

★ Order "Master Your DESTINY With Vastu" now to make the most of your Health, Relationships, Career, & Money by unlocking the Power of Directions.

<u>Check Out My Best Selling Books Here:</u>

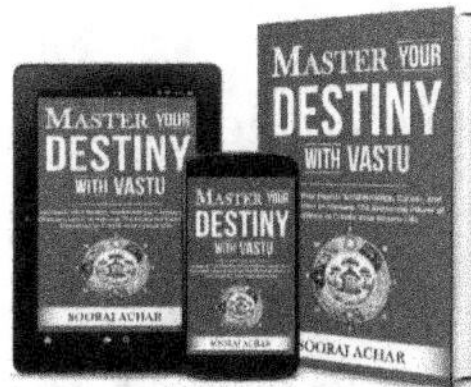

1. Master Your
DESTINY With Vastu

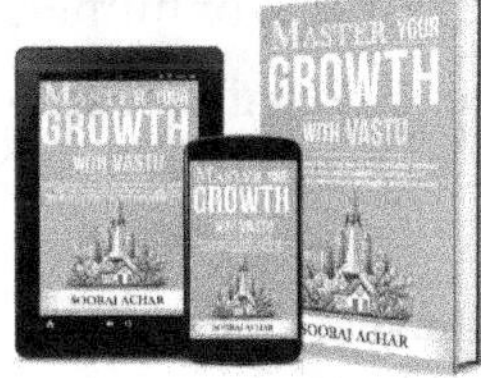

2. Master Your
GROWTH With Vastu

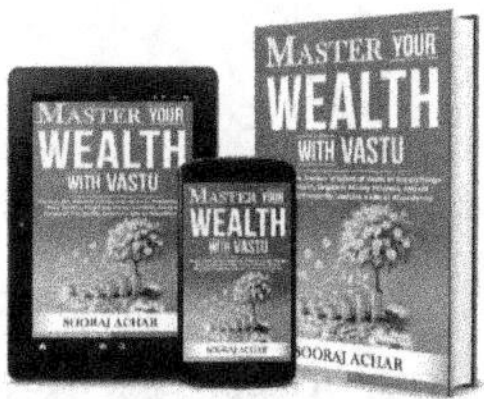

3. Master Your WEALTH
With Vastu

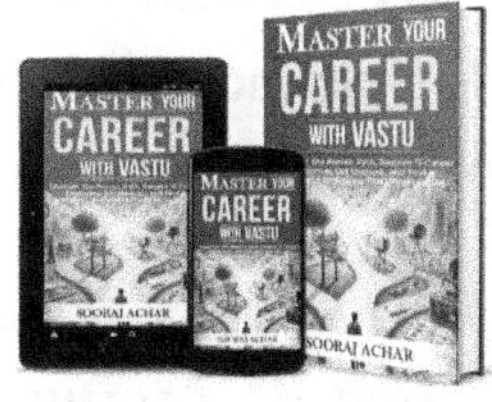

4. Master Your CAREER
With Vastu

<u>Series-3</u>: <u>The Ultimate Self-Healing</u> <u>Mastery</u>

Embark on a transformative expedition with 'The Ultimate Self-Healing Mastery,' a soul-stirring collection designed to illuminate the path to self-discovery, healing, and fearlessness. Each book is a profound exploration of fundamental aspects of human existence, guiding readers toward a purposeful, holistic, and fearless life.

1. Discover Your Life Purpose: Reveal Your True Calling

Uncover the secrets to a fulfilling life in 'Discover Your Life Purpose.' Illuminating the essence of your being, this book takes you on a profound journey to reveal your true calling. Master the art of purposeful living, radiate enduring joy, and align your actions with your life's deeper meaning. Through insightful practices and wisdom, you'll embark on a transformative odyssey to live a life that resonates with authenticity.

Key Themes: Life Purpose, Joyful Living, Authenticity

2. The Alchemy of Healing: Master Ancient Hawaiian Technique

In 'The Alchemy of Healing,' delve into the ancient Hawaiian wisdom that transcends time. Crush negative emotions, unravel subconscious patterns, and embark on a journey of self-healing for a holistic lifestyle. This book is a guide to harnessing the power within, using age-old techniques to restore balance, foster well-being, and tap into the alchemy that transforms challenges into opportunities for growth.

Key Themes: Ancient Healing, Emotional Wellness, Self-Healing

3. The Fear of Death: Conquer Mortality Anxiety, Live a Fearless Life

Confront the universal fear in 'The Fear of Death.' Recognize the human fears surrounding mortality, and transcend anxiety by embracing death as a natural part of life's journey. This book provides profound insights into conquering fears, living fearlessly, and understanding the deeper spiritual dimensions of existence. Gain wisdom to navigate life with courage, appreciating the transient nature of our earthly sojourn.

Key Themes: Fearlessness, Death Acceptance, Spiritual Wisdom

The Unifying Thread:

Each book in 'The Ultimate Self-Healing Mastery' is a standalone guide, yet together they form a cohesive narrative of personal growth, healing, and spiritual enlightenment. Authored by experts in their respective fields, these volumes offer a holistic approach to living—a roadmap to self-realization, emotional well-being, and a fearless embrace of life's profound mysteries.

Why Read the Trilogy?

Holistic Transformation: Embark on a journey that addresses the core aspects of your existence—purpose, healing, and fearlessness.

Expert Guidance: Benefit from the insights of experts who blend ancient wisdom with modern understanding to guide you toward a more meaningful and joyful life.

Practical Wisdom: Each book is a practical guide, filled with exercises, techniques, and profound teachings that can be applied in daily life.

Life-Altering Perspectives: Gain transformative perspectives on life purpose, healing practices, and the fear of death, allowing you to navigate challenges with resilience and grace.

Experience the synergy of purpose, healing, and fearlessness—the essence of 'The Ultimate Self-Healing Mastery.' This series is not just a collection of books; it's a transformative odyssey inviting you to explore the depths of your being and awaken to the infinite possibilities that life unfolds.

<u>Check Out My Best Selling Books Here:</u>

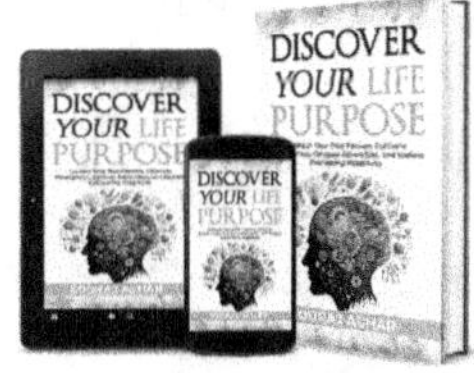

1. Discover Your Life Purpose

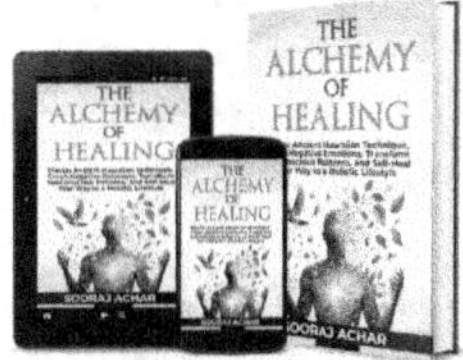

2. The Alchemy Of Healing

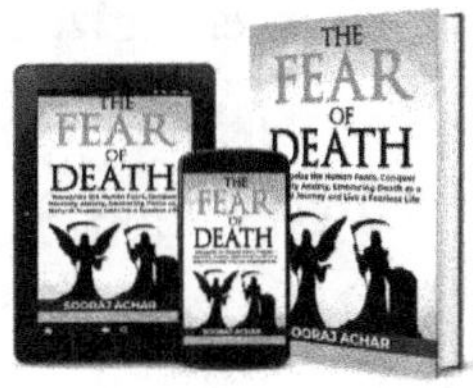

3. The Fear of Death

<u>Series-4</u>: <u>Energize Your Mind, Body & Soul</u>

Embark on a transformative journey of self-discovery, inner balance, and empowered living with the 'Energize Your Life Trilogy.' This compelling series unveils profound insights and practical wisdom to help you attain holistic well-being, align with your life's purpose, and cultivate the energy needed for a harmonious and fulfilling existence.

1. The Art of Balancing YIN-YANG Energy: Discover the Secret to Energized Living

Uncover the ancient wisdom of balancing YIN-YANG energy in 'The Art of Balancing YIN-YANG Energy.' This book is your guide to attaining wholeness, finding inner equilibrium, and experiencing serenity in your everyday existence. Learn the secrets of Chinese philosophy and energy balance to lead an energized life filled with vitality and peace. Discover practices to harmonize opposing forces, fostering a sense of completeness and tranquility.

Key Themes: Energy Balance, Wholeness, Serenity

2. The 7 Energy Needs: Discover the 7 Keys to Personal Fulfillment

In 'The 7 Energy Needs,' explore the keys to personal fulfillment and emotional well-being. Align your needs with your goals, master the art of balancing vital energies, and unlock the secrets to a harmonious life. This book provides a comprehensive framework for understanding and fulfilling your core energy needs, empowering you to lead a life rich in purpose, joy, and fulfillment.

Key Themes: Personal Fulfillment, Emotional Well-Being, Harmonious Life

3. The Power of ONE QUESTION: Master the Art of Smart Questioning

Ignite your journey to greatness with 'The Power of ONE QUESTION.' This book is a game-changer, offering insights into the art of smart questioning. Revolutionize your thinking, enhance decision-making, and supercharge your life and career by asking the right questions. Uncover the transformative power of focused inquiry and learn to navigate life's complexities with clarity, purpose, and a profound sense of direction.

Key Themes: Smart Questioning, Decision-Making, Journey to Greatness

The Unifying Thread:

The 'Energize Your Mind, Soul & Body' seamlessly weaves together the threads of ancient wisdom, modern psychology, and practical strategies. Each book stands as a beacon, guiding readers toward a more balanced, purposeful, and empowered life. The trilogy is designed to be both a comprehensive roadmap and a practical toolkit for individuals seeking a holistic approach to well-being and personal development.

Why Read the Trilogy?

1. **Holistic Well-Being:** Dive into a series that addresses the various dimensions of your well-being, from energy balance and emotional fulfillment to smart questioning and decision-making.

2. **Practical Wisdom:** Each book is crafted with practical exercises, actionable insights, and transformative practices that can be integrated into your daily life.

3. **Personal Empowerment:** Gain the tools and knowledge needed to take charge of your energy, align with your purpose, and make informed decisions that propel you toward greatness.

4. **Ancient Wisdom, Modern Application:**

Discover the timeless principles of ancient philosophies and see how they can be applied in the context of contemporary living.

Embark on a journey of self-mastery, inner harmony, and empowered living with the '**Energize Your Mind, Body & Soul**.' Let this series be your guide as you explore the depths of your potential and unlock the secrets to a more vibrant, purposeful, and harmonious life.

Check Out My Best Selling Books Here:

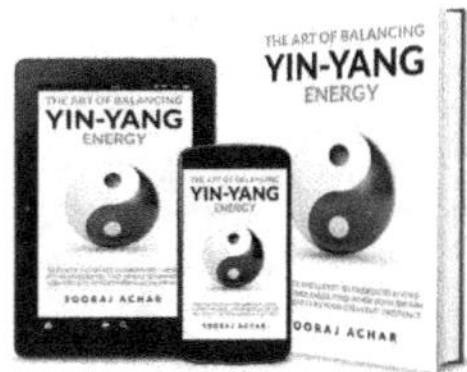

1. The Art of Balancing YIN-YANG Energy

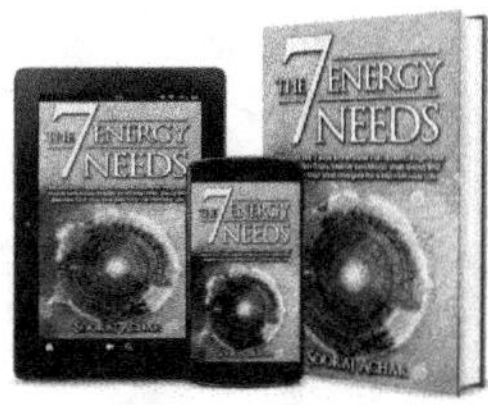

2. The 7 Energy Needs

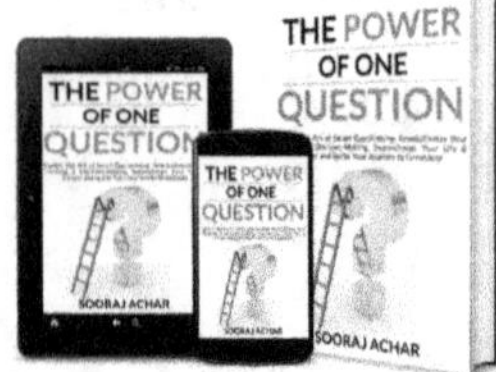

3. The Power Of ONE Question

Series-5: LIFE-MASTERY Bundle

From Book 1: **"Master Your DESTINY & NAME-SPELLING With Numerology"** takes you on an enlightening journey into the mystical world of numerology, where the power of numbers shapes the fabric of our destiny. In this comprehensive guide, author Sooraj Achar unravels the secrets behind the numbers that influence your life, offering profound insights into the science of numerology.

In This Book, You'll Discover:

1. Unlock Your Destiny: Explore the ancient science of numerology and unravel the mysteries of numbers that shape your life.

2. Name Spelling Mastery: Delve into the profound impact of name spelling on your destiny, discovering the hidden meanings within the letters.

3. Numerology Basics: Understand the core principles of numerology, from birthdate analysis to decoding the vibrations in your name.

4. Transformative Power: Witness real-life

examples showcasing the significant shifts that occur when altering the arrangement of letters in your name.

5. Personal Year Number Insights: Navigate the various phases of your life with wisdom by understanding the influence of your Personal Year Number.

6. Destiny Number Revelation: Calculate your Destiny Number to gain insights into your life's purpose, talents, and challenges, empowering informed decision-making.

7. Practical Tools: Engage in practical exercises, guided meditations, and interactive worksheets to apply numerology to your daily life.

8. Holistic Empowerment: Combine ancient wisdom with modern insights to create a holistic guide that empowers you to take charge of your destiny.

9. Transformative Journey: Whether you're a beginner or an experienced practitioner, embark on a journey of self-discovery, empowerment, and manifesting your fullest potential.

10. Illuminate Your Path: Decode the mysteries surrounding your name and birthdate, mastering your destiny through the profound wisdom of numerology.

11. Your Journey Begins Now: "Master Your DESTINY & NAME-SPELLING With Numerology" is your transformative tool for self-discovery and empowerment. Take the first step towards unlocking the secrets of your destiny.

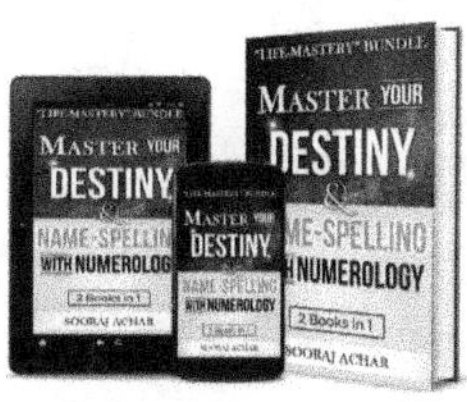

1. Master Your DESTINY & NAME-SPELLING With Numerology

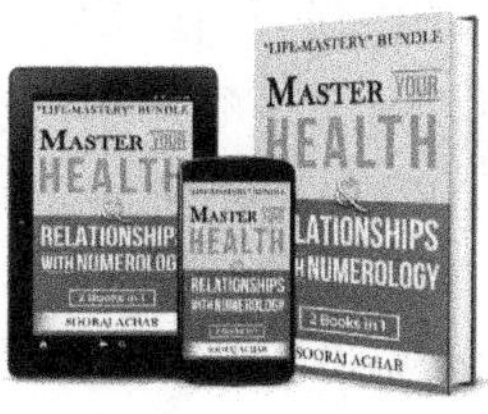

2. Master Your HEALTH & RELATIONSHIPS With Numerology

TESTIMONIALS

These are a few feedbacks from my clients across different parts of the world. Kindly go through their reviews to understand how Numerology and Vastu helped them.

1. Ekta Gupta – Kolkata, India

"2021 is a difficult year for me. I have consulted a few numerologists. I have received vague answers and complicated solutions. I'm new to numerology. Charges were expensive. Sooraj is a good and kind soul. He is very patient with me. He answered all my questions. I had 1000 questions. More ever he helped me to find a business name with no extra charges. I'm grateful to him. With your help, I'm sorted out with my business name. I had a lot of

anxiety about it. I'm confident now. Sooraj is a helpful soul. He is patient and explains if one has questions. He doesn't rush into closing the job. You can consult him easily. I am going to recommend him to newbies like me. He is not going to cheat you or misguide you".

2. Neetu Ganglani - Stanley, Hongkong

"Hello Sooraj, I can't thank you enough. At the age of 45, I could find an ideal life partner for myself. And my compatibility with the boy I like. Got to know our strengths and weaknesses. Your suggestions helped me to find the right life partner. You have a bright future. Good luck"

3. R Lensly Kwaimani - Solomon Islands, Oceania

"Dear friend, glad I came across you. My daughter Felinda Kwaimani is sick for a long time and I was very much worried. Thank you for giving suggestions and guidance".

4. Seham Shabhir - Talagang, Pakistan

"You're one of the best numerologists...your predictions are correct...you are a very humble person...you gave answers to all of my questions in detail ... I'm very thankful to you. Ur remedies prove very helpful for me. He is the very best numerologist... I recommend him for all.. u should consult him to get rid of your problems..his remedies work like a magic"

5. Naveen Kumar - Bengaluru, India

"Sooraj is a gem as a human and as a professional. Before approaching Sooraj, I have enquired and got inputs from other numerologists and I did some research as well. I Was not satisfied with the answers provided by them and most of them were behind fees, even after paying for the consultation they charge extra for clarifying doubts. However, Sooraj was awesome in client satisfaction and the way he follows up with the client for providing suggestions. He

takes the initiative to follow up and provide the best solutions and describes the reason for the input. I definitely suggest Sooraj to anyone who is looking for start-up business names or anything related to numerology. He has a good amount of knowledge and patience to answer all my queries".

6. Sneha S - Karnataka, India

"Hi Sooraj, it's a great prediction starting from Personality Traits to our Abroad Opportunities to future achievements. Everything is perfectly predicted with correct proof and explanations which help us to understand our lives better and take steps accordingly to numerology. Everyone are curious to know more about their life just to know when, how & what situations they will come across and how they need to overcome everything. Thanks a lot, Sooraj, for the best Numerology Prediction which helped us to understand ourselves better".

7. Aditya S - Mumbai, India

"Sooraj, your numerology predictions are brilliant and accurate. Your Suggestions helped me find out whether my current job is suitable for me or not. I would suggest people consult you in due course of time".

8. M Nabanita - West Bengal, India

"Hi Sooraj, it's helpful and gives me a quick idea and help. Thank you so much for being there. It helped me to understand my situation It helps in my career and marriage. The information is good".

9. N Naresh – Bangalore, India

"Hello Sooraj, it was satisfactory. Can decide further based on the info shared & also can see positive outcomes looking forward to checking how it works".

10. Harishchandra Dnyaneshwar Deshmukh – Delhi, India

"Hi sir, Padhai puri nahi kar paya, 11 k salary he, Stable nahi hu life me, Business success nahi milta. Thank u sir for sharing my report and helping me understand my strengths and weaknesses".

AUTHOR PROFILE

Follow **the Author's Profile Page** to get updates on all his books: **https://amazon.com/author/sooraj_achar**

Grab your **Free Gift** if you missed it: **https://gift.sooraj-achar.com/**

Please Leave Your **Valuable Review** here: **"The Alchemy of Healing"**

For 1-to-1 consultation, scan the **QR code** or contact: **connect@soorajachar.com**

Follow the **Author's BookBub** Profile: **BookBub Author Profile**

Stay Connected to the **Author's Social Media Handles** below:

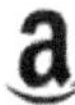

https://amzn.to/3CgQHF9

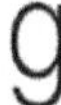

https://medium.com/@soorajachar99

https://bit.ly/3M7gIu2

instagram.com/psychology_of_numberz/

https://bit.ly/3dO6aDh

https://bit.ly/3LXBTyz

https://bit.ly/3E9vKxc

DISCLAIMER

This book is for educational purposes only. Readers acknowledge that the author does not render legal, financial, medical, or professional advice. The content within this book has been derived from various sources. Please consult a licensed professional before attempting any techniques outlined in this book.

By reading this document, the reader agrees that under no circumstances is the author responsible for any direct or indirect losses incurred as a result of the use of the information contained within this document, including but not limited to errors, omissions, or inaccuracies.

Adherence to all applicable laws and regulations, including international, federal, state, and local governing professional licensing, business practices, advertising, and all other jurisdictions, is the sole responsibility of the purchaser or reader.

Neither the author nor the publisher assumes any responsibility or liability whatsoever on behalf of the purchaser or reader of these materials. Any perceived slight of any individual or organization is purely unintentional.